THE EVERYTHING®
Tantric Sex Book

Dear Reader,

You are busy. Trust me, I know. But I took time to write this book, and you took time to read it, because we are perceptive enough to know that something is missing in our lives, despite our best efforts to cram every possible thing into a twenty-four-hour day.

What is this missing element? Calmness. Bliss. Contentment. If you are like most people, you are so caught up in the "rat race" and pursuing success (however you envision it) that you don't take enough time to nurture your spirit and your soul.

By learning how to achieve balance within yourself—and with your partner, as well as the world around you—you can lead a life of happiness and harmony. And since personal relationships are often the first casualties of a busy life, picking up a few tricks to spice up your sex life can strengthen your intimate bond with your partner. Bottom line: I think your pursuit of Tantra will bring light and sunshine into your life in all sorts of magical ways.

I hope this book will help you find spiritual bliss and personal contentment. Not to mention, a hot and passionate sex life.

—*Bobbi Dempsey*

The EVERYTHING® Series

Editorial

Publisher	Gary M. Krebs
Director of Product Development	Paula Munier
Managing Editor	Laura M. Daly
Associate Copy Chief	Sheila Zwiebel
Acquisitions Editor	Kerry Smith
Development Editor	Brett Palana-Shanahan
Production Editor	Casey Ebert

Production

Director of Manufacturing	Susan Beale
Production Project Manager	Michelle Roy Kelly
Prepress	Erick DaCosta
	Matt LeBlanc
Interior Layout	Heather Barrett
	Brewster Brownville
	Colleen Cunningham
	Jennifer Oliveira
Cover Design	Erin Alexander
	Stephanie Chrusz
	Frank Rivera

THE
EVERYTHING®
TANTRIC SEX
BOOK

Learn meditative, spontaneous,
and intimate lovemaking

Bobbi Dempsey
Technical Review by Al Link and Pala Copeland
Founders, 4 Freedoms (*www.tantra-sex.com*)

Adams Media
Avon, Massachusetts

To my beloved readers—may you find balance, love, and bliss.

An Everything® Series Book.
Everything® and everything.com® are registered trademarks of F+W Publications, Inc.

Published by Adams Media, an F+W Publications Company
57 Littlefield Street, Avon, MA 02322 U.S.A.
www.adamsmedia.com

ISBN-10: 1-59869-326-3
ISBN-13: 978-1-59869-326-3

Printed in the United States of America.

J   I   H   G   F   E   D   C   B   A

Library of Congress Cataloging-in-Publication Data
Dempsey, Bobbi.
The everything tantric sex book / Bobbi Dempsey with
Al Link and Pala Copeland.
p. cm. — (Everything series)
ISBN-13: 978-1-59869-326-3 (pbk.)
ISBN-10: 1-59869-326-3 (pbk.)
1. Sex instruction. 2. Sex—Religious aspects—Tantrism.
3. Man-woman relationships. I. Link, Al. II. Copeland, Pala.
III. Title.
HQ31.D419 2007
306.77—dc22   2007010854

Interior Illustrations by Kathie Kelleher

This book is available at quantity discounts for bulk purchases.
For information, please call 1-800-289-0963.

Contents

Acknowledgments

I would like to extend my sincere thanks to the Tantric experts, teachers, and practitioners who generously offered their advice and input for this book. Their insight and wisdom is greatly appreciated. Also, much gratitude to the many ancient gurus who practiced and preserved their mystical beliefs even under great duress and prejudice, ensuring this spiritual art would live on throughout the centuries.

Top Ten Reasons Why You Should Practice Tantric Sex

1. Tantra helps you connect with the universe and the higher power, leading to spiritual healing and enlightenment.

2. You will be a happier person. For most people, Tantra brings a sense of peace and joy that may have been missing in their lives.

3. Your orgasms will become much stronger, more satisfying, occur more frequently, and last longer than they did before.

4. You will rediscover your own body.

5. Relatedly, you will also see your partner's body in a whole new light. Most likely, you will find exciting new spots that you previously neglected or overlooked.

6. Tantra stresses the importance of balance, which brings an overall sense of calm into one's life.

7. The incredibly powerful intimate bond you develop with your partner will benefit both of you. The connection you build through Tantra will make your union stronger and more fulfilling.

8. Your fitness level will greatly improve. Many of the techniques associated with Tantra—yoga, Kegel exercises, etc.—can have great fitness benefits such as muscle strengthening and toning. Bottom line: it does a body good.

9. You will have some fun shopping trips. Hitting the stores in search of perfect items for your sacred space and fun toys for your bedroom adventures sure beats grocery shopping!

10. Everybody loves good sex! And your partner will be thrilled at the new moves you pull out of your sexual bag of tricks.

Introduction

▶ CONGRATULATIONS. By making the decision to check out this book, you have taken an important first step on an entirely new journey in your life—embarking on a path that can lead you to a special place where you feel both ultimate peace and unbridled passion.

Peace and passion. A highly desirable combination—and a state of being that many people pursue, but few are able to successfully achieve. You will be following a path created for you by Tantric trailblazers of ancient times. By heeding the wisdom of the past, you will be paving the way for your blissful new future.

Let's face it: If having a powerful and fulfilling intimate connection were as easy as inserting Tab A into Slot B, everybody would be in a constant state of bedroom bliss. Instead, many people find themselves feeling frustrated and disappointed in their personal relationships, constantly searching for the elusive key to ecstasy. They may go from one unsatisfying relationship to another, never seeming to find what they need. Eventually, they reach a point of reluctant acceptance and resign themselves to the fact that "this is all there is." They abandon all hope of ever having more—more passion, more happiness, and more spiritual peace.

But it gives me great pleasure to tell you it doesn't have to be that way. No matter what your background or current situation, you too can have balance and happiness in your life. You can eliminate stress and negative energy from your life. And, finally, you can reach new heights of passion with your partner. As a bonus, you will also learn how to have a loving, blissful existence with the world around you—and understand how to achieve peace and acceptance within yourself.

With the help of ancient gurus and the sexual and spiritual secrets they dedicated themselves to protecting, you will first learn how to attain harmony in your life, which will then pave the way toward a completely fulfilling love life.

There is an old saying that the brain is the most important sex organ. There is a lot of truth to that—although you must also include two other critical elements: the heart and soul. So rather than just throwing you into a menu of various exciting sex positions, this book first takes you on a journey toward a more content and enlightened soul. You will learn about the history of Tantra, including the ancient traditions that gurus carefully preserved and passed down to trusted students. You will also discover the differences between the various types of Tantra, which can help you decide which path is right for you.

Before just jumping into bed with a bottle of massage oil (and, ideally, a partner) you will learn the importance of touch and why you first need to establish a powerful intimate connection. You will become skilled at creating the all-important sacred space for love, and find out why those pre-intercourse rituals and routines are so important.

You will learn how to prepare yourself—mentally, emotionally, and physically—for the most passionate encounters you may ever have. Realizing that spiritual and emotional factors play a big part in physical pleasure, you will learn techniques for establishing and/or strengthening an intimate bond with the special person in your life. Once you have completed that goal, you will discover the key to the most passionate—maybe even magical—sex of your life.

In pursuing Tantric enlightenment, you will also discover a new and exciting network of like-minded people. You will find yourself with many new friends who share your interest in self-improvement and higher consciousness.

Perhaps most importantly, you will learn the importance of treating yourself and your partner with the love, respect, and adoration that you deserve. You will learn to expect the treatment befitting a god or goddess, while also bestowing appropriate treatment upon your partner.

By employing ancient Tantric approaches and attitudes, you will open yourself up to new levels of passion and spiritual peace that will cast a glow of positive energy over your entire universe.

Welcome to an exciting phase of your life. Your future is bright and radiant with joy. Embrace this new beginning and revel in the spiritual awakening it brings you. May you enjoy total bliss in your life—and your love.

Chapter 1

Tantric Sex 101

You may be familiar with the saying, "everything old is new again," and that's definitely true when it comes to the art of sensual pleasure. Tantric sex is among the oldest (if not *the* oldest) of all the sensual arts. Yet it is recently becoming more popular than ever. More and more people are becoming fans of Tantra and the positive effects it can have on their love life. Read on and discover how an ancient philosophy can spice up the sex life of a modern person like you.

What Does Tantra Mean?

The word *Tantra* is Sanskrit for "weave" or "woven together." Sometimes it is also translated to mean "to expand" or "to liberate." It is a system of beliefs and traditions—based on the art of consciousness—dating back to ancient times. The roots of Tantra are obscure. Some say the practice dates back many thousands of years to early goddess worship. Tantra became extremely popular in India in the eighth through twelfth centuries, working its way across the country and even making its way to rural villages.

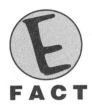

FACT

Sanskrit is a classical language used in Hinduism and Buddhism. Some people believe it is the world's oldest language. It is one of India's twenty-two official languages, but has mainly become a language for research scholars. It is not used as a common form of communication.

The term *Tantra* has been used loosely over the years, applied to several different bodies of beliefs—mostly those based on Hindu and Buddhist traditions celebrating the union of what appear to be opposites. In other words, celebrating the union of masculine and feminine, positive and negative, etc., in order to transcend the perceived separateness and regain the actual oneness of reality. Tantra also involves the idea of using the union of man and woman—meaning intercourse—as a route to a divine place. In some cases, intercourse was seen as a path to God or a higher spiritual universe.

A main tenet of the Tantra philosophy is that all aspects of life, all living things and of creation, are special and sacred. Simply put, it's the basic idea of creating "heaven on earth" and viewing yourself as a god or goddess. Using Tantric teachings, people learn to form a spiritual connection with everything and everyone around them.

People who practice the traditional art of Tantra are called *Tantrics* (also *Tantrikas* or *Tantricas*). In traditional Tantra, Tantrics would spend years studying under a guru and would engage in elaborate, often time-consuming, rituals and exercises to perfect their skills and sharpen their minds and spirits.

The Basic Idea

Tantra involves many different beliefs and practices, but there is one common theme. In all practices, there is an emphasis on the joining of two seemingly opposite life forces—male and female, yin and yang, dark and light, hot and cold, etc.—to create one powerful force leading to higher consciousness. Basically, by joining these two halves, you make a whole, which leads to spiritual (and sensual) bliss.

It's All about Unity

The basic principle of Tantra is unity. That can be expressed in many forms. It could be unity with the world around you, or unity of spirit, which brings peace and clarity, or when related to sex, the unity of man and woman to bring about the ultimate pleasure and fulfillment. Once you achieve the desired unity, you reach a higher consciousness and connect with a divine place. (In traditional Tantra, this usually involved a connection with a god, a creator, an ultimate being, or some other deity, but today it is often interpreted to mean a place of complete bliss.)

The Ancient Approach

In ancient Hindu times, the Tantra approach to sex involved using meditation combined with nonorgasmic sensual activities, resulting in spiritual bliss. This technique involved activating and stimulating the energy centers (the chakras, which will be discussed in detail in Chapter 13), each of which played an important role in helping participants pursue their ultimate spiritual destination.

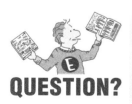

QUESTION?

What is sacred sex?
When the techniques of Tantra are applied to sensual acts, this is sometimes referred to as "sacred sex." This term is used to refer to any sexual experience that helps a person attain a stronger connection with the universe or a higher power.

Shiva and Shakti

When discussing Tantra and the idea of unity, it is necessary to include Shiva and Shakti, who represent masculine and feminine archetypes in Hindu symbolism. Shiva, the male, is pure consciousness; Shakti, the female, is the power of creation—she's the life force energy that combines with his power of thought to manifest the physical world. One cannot exist without the other, as the two are inseparable and it takes both powers working in harmony to keep the universe functioning (more on Shiva and Shakti in Chapter 3).

Tantra's Bad Reputation

For a long time, Tantric practices were frowned upon in many regions of the world (to a lesser extent, this bias still exists today). This was largely due to myths and misconceptions surrounding Tantra. People in the scientific community wrongly believed that Tantra was based on superstition. Also, some of the traditional Tantric rituals—often marked by chanting, dancing, sacrificial rites (including human sacrifices), images of gods and goddesses, and other mystical/religious elements—made people think of a cult, or witchcraft, or black magic. But perhaps the most important opposition came from those in power, who disliked Tantra's philosophy of freedom and openness, perhaps fearing it would make people too rebellious and independent.

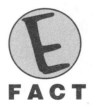

FACT

Modern Tantra is not a religion, although it focuses on spiritual enlightenment. You can practice Tantric techniques regardless of your religious faith. You do not need to renounce your current religion to practice Tantra. Ideally, Tantra should enhance your established beliefs, not replace them.

Even today, some people prejudge Tantra as being too "New Age" or obscure, usually because they haven't taken the time to learn about Tantric beliefs or understand the principles behind them. Perhaps people also mistakenly believe that Tantra is a religion—and therefore they cannot observe its teachings while adhering to their own particular religious beliefs.

Why Westerners Need It

People today may be more "free" about sex as far as discussing it openly and feeling comfortable with their sexuality, but for the most part they are still not nearly as enlightened when it comes to sex as they may like to think.

Sexual Enlightenment

A lot of people today confuse promiscuous behavior with sexual enlightenment. This couldn't be further from the truth. Just because you have a multitude of partners, this does not mean you are sexually enlightened. In fact, many followers of Tantra are advocates of monogamy and committed relationships. The whole idea behind Tantric sex is to make the experience more fulfilling, both physically and emotionally, allowing you to form a bond with your partner that's stronger than ever. As a result, sex is infinitely more pleasurable and never gets boring, even if you've been with the same partner for a long time. By learning to make the experience itself more enjoyable, you eliminate the need to continue to search for new partners to keep things exciting. Essentially, by fulfilling the spiritual aspect of sex, as a higher power intended, the desire for multiple sex partners is decreased because the emotional void is filled.

Slow Things Down

In our fast-paced world, there's a tendency to focus on quick gratification and purely physical encounters. True, such quickie encounters can be satisfying in the short-term, but eventually you realize that you crave more. By slowing things down and focusing on forming a strong spiritual connection, you will have sensual encounters that will prove much more satisfying.

In addition, Tantra emphasizes relaxation, togetherness, creativity, and playfulness. These are all things that can come in handy for the busy people rushing through today's high-stress environment. Taking the time to smell the roses (or your partner's unique enchanting scent) can be a great way to escape the stresses and pressures of daily life.

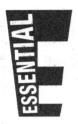

Western philosophy is generally concerned with the outer world—how to achieve success outside of one's self. Eastern philosophy teaches the importance of cultivating one's inner strength. That is, it teaches that success cannot be measured by outer achievements.

Embrace Emotions

In the West, there is a lot of emphasis on logic, reason, and linear thought. In the East, however, there is intuition, belief, and circular thought. One teacher described the difference in perceptions like this: The westerner sees the world, while the easterner feels the world.

Yet, in the West, throughout history so much emphasis has been placed on logic that the feeling is missing. Westerners are more and more interested in getting control over emotions rather than the "let it out" approach and deep-relaxation techniques.

Ideas of Eastern and Western spirituality generally suggest that the East is passive while the West is active. In analyzing the different schools of Tantra, we can see that this is not always true. This "live it" aspect of Eastern spirituality appeals to many westerners who wish to experience spirituality and are no longer content simply contemplating it.

Is It All about Sex?

There are many misconceptions when it comes to the subjects of sex and Tantra. The most common, is that *Tantra* means "sex." While it's true that Tantra principles can greatly enrich and enhance your sex life, that's just one aspect of a much broader way of life. In reality, Tantra is a large philosophy encompassing many areas of life, and sex is only one small part of that. But since sex is—in the Western world—the most well known (and, arguably, the most titillating) part of Tantra, it gets the most attention.

In Tantra, desires are expected and embraced. They are viewed as a natural part of being human. They are to be encouraged and learned from. Desire becomes a vehicle for spiritual awakening. This is very different from what the Western approach teaches.

Tantra beliefs and teachings can help you improve all aspects of your life. This philosophy can help you take a fresh new look at everything around you. You will learn to view all of creation as a spiritual, heavenly universe—and to view yourself as a god or goddess inhabiting that universe.

A Tantra Guru Weighs In

Al Link and his partner Pala Copeland have been Tantric sex practitioners since 1987 and teachers since 1997. They are the authors of *Soul Sex: Tantra for Two* and several other books on the subject. Al shares his thoughts on Tantra's connection to sex:

> *There is an interesting split in the Tantric community about the meaning and significance of Tantra sacred sex practices. At one extreme, there are those teachers who claim that sex has nothing to do with the "'true" or "pure" spiritual Tantra. At the other extreme there are those who believe that enhanced sexuality is all that Tantra is about. There is also a middle position, such as ours, which maintains that in its spiritual dimension, as a vehicle leading practitioners toward full enlightenment, that all aspects of life in a body are sacred and to be celebrated, indeed that nothing is to be denied or excluded. This includes a healthy joyous sexuality, a sacred sexuality.*
>
> *Our teaching is that sex is good, pleasure is good, sex is sacred, and sacred sex is definitely a spiritual aspect of Tantra. Sex doesn't bring one to an enlightened consciousness, nor do other Tantric practices such as meditation, ceremony, ritual, prayer, and physical and psychological techniques such as relaxation, breathing, visualization, chanting, mantras, yantras, mandalas, mudras, and so on. It's not the activity itself that brings one to an awakened state—practices are simply vehicles to help one become clear, focused, and present in the eternal now.*

The Broader Picture

Tantric teachings usually combine yoga, meditation, breathing exercises, workshops, written materials—all of this in addition to information on the sexual aspect of Tantra.

However, obviously, you picked up this book because you have an interest in Tantra as it relates to sex specifically, so this book will focus most of the information on that part of the Tantra philosophy. But it is important to at least briefly touch on the ways that Tantra can affect your entire life. The first and most basic way? Tantra can make you feel more peaceful, spiritually balanced, and emotionally fulfilled. This fulfillment improves all aspects of your life as a whole, and in turn, also makes your love life better. After all, when your life in general is happy, balanced, and fulfilling, your sex life can't help but reap the benefits.

Personal Benefits

Tantra can have many benefits to an individual. Tantra in its traditional form as a true spiritual practice holds a very important place in the lives of the practitioners. It creates calmness and awareness. Tantra makes change possible. It spurs spiritual evolution by awakening energies within you that would otherwise remain dormant.

Here in the West people learn to suppress desire, as it is often associated with weakness and sin. They are taught to be strong and self-denying. This can cause more damage than good to a person's well being. By denying yourself experiences that may be enriching or that may further your spiritual quest simply because they are desires, you create repressed emotions and regrets, leading to a host of other complications. You will eventually begin to feel unfulfilled and will grow resentful of constantly being forced to stifle your desires. That is why it is better to learn about yourself, your strengths and weakness, through your desires, thereby becoming a more whole, fuller individual. Bottom line: Embracing and heeding your desires, rather than opposing them, can be a very good thing.

Additionally, the East considers the individual as part of the integrated whole. The West traditionally sees the individual as separated from the whole. More and more seekers are in need of feelings of unity and connection, not division and separation. Tantra can provide that feeling of unity.

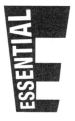

Many westerners feel empty after dedicating their lives to the outer world. Eastern religions and philosophies provide them with an answer. Philosophies such as those connected to Tantra can provide people with a feeling of fulfillment that they can't get from material things.

Other Benefits of Tantra

Aside from improving your life overall and enriching your sex life, there are lots of other ways you can benefit from studying the Tantra philosophies and incorporating them into your daily routine. By becoming more conscious of your body's well-being—spiritually, emotionally, and physically—you will find that you start taking better care of yourself. The meditation and breathing exercises connected to Tantra are great stress relievers—as are the yoga exercises, which also can do wonders for your body physically.

In addition, a core principle of Tantra is enriching your relationship with those around you, and strengthening the bond you have with loved ones.

Lastly, by studying the Tantric emphasis on higher consciousness, you will experience personal growth and spiritual evolution that will benefit all facets of your life. So, while you may initially be interested in studying Tantra for the sexual benefits, you can apply the lessons you learn to virtually all other aspects of your life, making your entire world a much better place to be!

Neo-Tantra: What It Is and Isn't

Neo-Tantra is a term used to refer to the modern-day version of Tantra. It is also known as "New Age" Tantra or "Western Tantra." Neo-Tantra practitioners don't adhere to all of the traditional Tantric beliefs and techniques. For example, many Neo-Tantra fans don't view all sexual encounters as a ritual, as is common with traditional Tantra. That is not to say that one practice is better or more respectable than the other, but rather that they are different and that the terms are not interchangeable.

There are many characteristics that set westernized Tantra apart from traditional Tantra. Take the guru, for example. In traditional Tantra, the guru is the ultimate authority and treated with utmost respect. This spiritual master is essential to assuring a positive and enriching spiritual experience. In traditional Tantra, the principal interests are the guru-disciple relationship and ritual discipline.

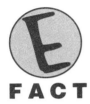

FACT

There is significant difference between Tantric and Neo-Tantric philosophy in regard to the importance placed on orgasm. For example, Buddhist Tantra views the orgasm as essentially an irrelevant event, as it is believed that this energy should be used toward spiritual awakening. In Neo-Tantra, however, the orgasm (albeit, often an enhanced or prolonged orgasm) is encouraged as a way to increase pleasure, both for the man and the woman.

In westernized Tantra, on the other hand, the guru is not an important figure, as each person in the relationship acts as the teacher. In westernized Tantra, both people in the relationship assume the position of the teacher and the transmitter of truth. Each person learns from the other and experiences spiritual truth through their union.

Neo-Tantra and Sex

In traditional Tantra, sex was seen as just one piece of the puzzle. The pure, traditional Tantra philosophy stressed total-body happiness—spiritually, physically, sexually, etc. With Neo-Tantra, however, sex takes center stage. Things like male multiple orgasm and female ejaculation—which are not really stressed in traditional Tantra—are given much more attention in the westernized version. Also, Neo-Tantra tends to stress the "G-spot orgasm," as opposed to the full-body orgasm of traditional Tantra. Many modern Tantra fans are primarily interested in the sexual aspects of the philosophy. They may know almost nothing about the background and lessons of Tantra—they simply want to learn how to use its techniques to improve their sex life.

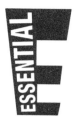

In Neo-Tantra, couples generally use the ideas of spiritual peace and other elements to enhance their relationship. Whereas with traditional Tantra it's somewhat the opposite—the goal is to use the relationship as a tool to attain higher levels of peace and consciousness.

Neo-Tantra brings sex into the light, making the practitioner more sexually aware. It gives you the opportunity to expand your limits of pleasure, to try new positions and techniques, and to delve deeper into intimacy. It helps you to have better, fuller orgasms and deeper, more meaningful communication in the bedroom. By bettering the quality of your intimate relationships, you better yourself, your partner, and those around you. Not to mention, every aspect of your life is bound to benefit when you achieve a greater sense of peace, balance, and harmony with the world.

In essence, Neo-Tantrics believe pleasure has spiritual value; pleasure is a path of spiritual practice. Neo-Tantra deals more with increasing intimacy, having better orgasms, and deepening relationships. Neo-Tantra can help fill a void that many people may feel in their personal lives. It adds a deeper dimension to one's sex life and therefore one's love life, and possibly even has the potential to affect one's outlook and lifestyle in general.

What Neo-Tantra Is Not

Neo-Tantra offers many benefits to those who follow its techniques, and is also a good way to introduce some Tantra beliefs to those who otherwise may not be willing or able to study Tantra. Still, it is important to note that Neo-Tantra is not the traditional, ancient version of Tantra. It is not "pure" Tantra. Indeed, many Tantra purists take a negative or critical view of Neo-Tantra. However, Neo-Tantra may be more attractive and suitable for many people in this modern age, especially in the United States. Many people just don't have the dedication or interest to study the traditional Tantra lessons. However, if you choose to study Neo-Tantra, it is much better to incorporate at least some of the Tantra teachings into your life as well, rather than none at all.

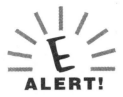

ALERT!

If you are interested in learning more about Neo-Tantra, there are plenty of groups, workshops, and related resources available. However, use caution and do your research. Some unethical and unsavory groups have taken to using the term *Neo-Tantra* as a way to lure unsuspecting people into "clubs" that are thinly disguised escort services or other objectionable endeavors.

Here's a little secret: Even if you start out only interested in learning about the sexual aspects of Tantra, you will almost inevitably learn about many other aspects of the philosophy. Ideally, this book will provide a blend of the best of both worlds—the sexual and sensual advice you want, but the spiritual and informative material that will also prove very helpful. And maybe once you read this book on Tantric sex, you will be inspired to do further research on the topic of traditional Tantric beliefs.

Tantra in the Modern World

Recently, there has been a renewed interest in Tantra—both the traditional type and the westernized variety—in the United States. Maybe that is because people today tend to be more sexually open and adventurous than in the past.

Westerners are generally more repressed and uptight about sex than people in other parts of the world. Sex in the West is often associated with sin. Until very recently, it had no place in spiritual or religious practices. This has made sex confining and at times even dark. Tantra and Neo-Tantra have provided westerners with a way to explore sexuality through spirituality. It has brought together these two realms that are really interconnected. Part of the reason that Neo-Tantra has been so successful is because it meets the needs of westerners everywhere. It fits in exactly where there is a gap that needs to be filled.

There is also a general interest in things viewed as "New Age," like yoga and meditation. Books on Tantra are selling in great numbers. There are countless Web sites on the topic, in addition to magazines, videos, and workshops. Today virtually everyone—no matter where he or she lives—has access to information about Tantra and the ability to discuss it openly and share knowledge with others.

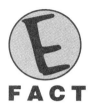

FACT

Tantra has become more well known (and more widely accepted) in the United States thanks to high-profile fans like the singer Sting and his wife Trudie Styler, who have openly raved about the benefits of Tantra in their relationship and sex life. Actor Woody Harrelson has also publicly discussed his experiences with Tantric sex.

Tantra Across the World

In various scattered regions of India, authentic traditional Tantra is still practiced by devoted followers. However, this is done mainly in secrecy. The gurus who teach Tantra are viewed as almost godlike, and the whole process is handled with extreme reverence. It definitely would not be discussed as openly or casually as it would be in the United States. Tibetan Tantra is also practiced by many native Tibetans in Tibetan Buddhist locations throughout Europe and America.

Chapter 2

History of Tantric Sex

Tantric sex is no fad or "flavor of the month" bedroom trend. It has actually been around for thousands of years. References to the Tantric sex principles and beliefs can be found in writings of early Buddhist teachers. But many couples today realize that Tantra can really give their bedroom activities a boost. This chapter will explore the history of Tantra and some of the groups and individuals who have helped formulate and preserve its traditions.

The Roots of Tantra

Tantra is an ancient body of beliefs that has been held sacred by many groups of people throughout history. It was a widespread practice in ancient India and Tibet. Its influence was also felt as Tantric ideas and practices spread to other regions such as Egypt and China. Tantra was very prevalent between the seventh and thirteenth centuries.

Tantra is a term that is most commonly used to refer to this philosophy of beliefs directed at forming a spiritual connection with the universe. The term also refers to the sacred writings related to those beliefs. However, other types of written Hindu documents—such as those related to scientific, medical, and astrological topics—are sometimes also referred to by the general term of *Tantras*.

It can be tricky to try and trace the history of Tantra because much of it is shrouded in secrecy. This was partly because it was misunderstood. Tantra was often perceived as involving sorcery or black magic. To the uninformed, casual observer of early times, it may have just looked and sounded like a lot of hocus-pocus. But Tantra was a private, personal practice that wasn't commonly discussed openly in public.

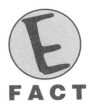

FACT

In ancient Hindu, the word *Tantra* often referred to the joining or connection of two forces. Sometimes sexual terms or depictions were used to illustrate this, but it often really had nothing to do with actually having sex.

In many cases, the teachings and traditions of Tantra were passed directly from guru to student verbally (sometimes with the help of nonwritten aids such as art, music, etc.), so there weren't a lot of written materials to be saved for posterity. This is unfortunate, as those early Tantric gurus probably had a lot of impressive wisdom to offer. Modern-day Tantrics could likely benefit greatly from the lessons these early pioneers could have shared. This scarcity of written records also makes it more difficult to pinpoint exact milestones in the evolution of this sacred art.

It is generally accepted that Tantra dates back at least 3,000 years, originating in India. Over the years, Tantra in various forms has also been practiced in many other areas of the world, including Tibet, China, and Korea.

Hindu Tantric Traditions

According to Hindu lore, the Tantras came from communications between Shiva and Shakti very long ago, probably at least 2000 B.C. or earlier. Some of these conversations were overheard and passed along from gurus to their students, and eventually were documented in written form.

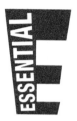

Some people believe the earliest roots of Tantra date all the way back to branches of Hinduism called *Shaktism* and *Shaivism*. These religions were based on the worship of Shakti and Shiva in their many forms.

Hindu and Buddhist Tantra both place an emphasis on rituals—specifically, rituals involving sex, food, and wine. Many of these rituals would also frequently involve dancing, music, and other forms of entertainment. (For more on rituals see Chapter 12.)

Tantric Buddhism

Tantric Buddhism (also known as "Tibetan Buddhism" or "Vajrayana") traces its roots to the teachings and life of Siddhartha Gautama, the Buddha, who was born in Nepal during the sixth century B.C. His beliefs centered around the idea of the "Middle Path"—meaning the philosophy of seeking enlightenment through balance and moderation. It is believed that Buddhist Tantra originated somewhere around the fourth century through a slow process in which teachings were passed down quietly from teacher to pupil. It most likely originated with the monks, and even once it spread to other parts of the population, some secret teachings were still reserved for monks alone. Tantric Buddhism gathered momentum by the eighth century and was even adopted by rulers during the period of Bengal's Pala dynasty (A.D. 750 to 1150).

Somewhere along the way Tantric Buddhism has also adopted elements of Bon, the indigenous religion of Tibet. As a result, this type of Buddhism has developed into a very distinctive form of the religion.

In Buddhist Tantra, it is believed that you can use sex to help you reach a state of bliss and supreme enlightenment. Followers are taught to revere the body and to indulge its sensual desires and impulses. This was a sharp contrast to the traditional branch of Buddhism, called Theravada, where strict discipline and self-denial are cardinal rules. Those who follow the Theravada doctrines generally live a very spartan, modest lifestyle, with little importance placed on materialistic pleasures, and spend a great deal of time on meditation. The ritual sex activities common in Tantric Buddhism are totally foreign (not to mention prohibited and frowned upon) to the followers of Theravada.

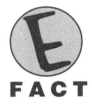

FACT

In traditional Buddhist Tantra, a sex partner was called a *karma mudra*. By contrast, a *jnana mudra* was a fantasy partner, one that was only "present" in the person's fantasy. Interestingly, jnana mudra is also a sacred Tantric hand gesture in which the hand is held at chest level and the index finger and thumb touch to form a circle while the other three fingers extend upward.

The sex rituals that were sometimes parts of Buddhist Tantra were large and elaborate, often involving anywhere from ten to fifty celebrants. It was an indulgent event, and not just in a sexual way. Celebrants often smoked cannabis, drank alcohol, and enjoyed a huge feast.

In addition to the sexual aspects, Tantric Buddhism was also seen as controversial because it essentially offered a shortcut to nirvana. In the more traditional types of Buddhism, it is believed that followers must study intently and dedicate themselves to their faith, cultivating their spiritual perfection over the course of several lifetimes. By contrast, Tantric Buddhism offered the ability to reach this state much more quickly, in less than a single lifetime.

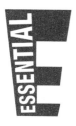

People are often surprised to learn that Buddhist Tantra can be traced back to early monasteries. It is believed that many of the founders of Buddhist Tantra were monks and others who felt compelled to rebel against the rigid rules and attitudes of the religious and spiritual leadership which were common in ancient times.

The Siddhas

The first significant Tantric-related records date back to the time of the Siddhas. *Siddha* is a Sanskrit term that refers to someone who had attained the status of a "grand master." In parts of India, a Siddha was believed to be an individual who had attained both spiritual and physical perfection, to the point where he had become immortal. There was a broad Siddha movement involving Hindu and Buddhist people that occurred as part of an era known as the "Pan-Indian Tantric Yoga Movement" beginning around the seventh century and continuing until around the eleventh century. The Tamil Siddhas were a specific religious group within that movement which originated in the southern region of India sometime around the eighth century. You might say the Tamil Siddhas were a rebel group. They were viewed by more conservative religious orders to be heretics, because the Tamil Siddhas practiced beliefs that were considered unorthodox and controversial for that time.

But the important thing from a historical viewpoint is that the Tamil Siddhas were among the first to put Tantric texts down on paper. However, they did not make their writings easy to understand. They used a lot of poetic verse, often in an ancient style, and also employed a lot of imagery and symbolism.

Tantra's Dark Period

Somewhere around the eighth century, Tantric practitioners were forced to go "underground" and practice their beliefs covertly, because Tantra was viewed as strange and perhaps connected to black magic. The sex rituals commonly associated with Tantra were also viewed as highly controversial during this time.

During a drawn-out period usually assumed to have been between the seventh and twelfth centuries, Muslims invaded India and enacted laws prohibiting many popular beliefs. Anyone caught following Tantric beliefs or practices could be executed during this period.

As a result of these and other occurrences, Tantric followers in India and other regions were forced to be very secretive about their actions for several centuries.

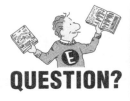

QUESTION?

What are left-handed and right-handed Tantras?
In some older writings about Tantra, believers are divided into two groups—left-handed and right-handed—based on the path the person took in following the Tantric teachings. Left-handed Tantras were the ones who regularly indulged in sensory pleasures and "vices," such as alcohol, meat, and sex, and incorporated these pleasures into their rituals. Right-handed Tantras had more self-control and were generally viewed to be more spiritually pure and disciplined. Right-handed Tantra did not include sexual acts.

Taoist Traditions

Taoism, a major Asian religion, has its own Tantra-like traditions. In fact these two philosophies can be confused because they have similar approaches to many topics. Certain forms of Taoism and Tantra are parallel, but the philosophies are not the same. Some Tantra-like traditions in Taoism include those based on the idea that you can harness the energy of the sexual reproductive drive (referred to as *jing*, or *ching*) and use it for better health and happiness. In Taoism, the primary goal of sex is not necessarily physical pleasure, but rather to promote longevity and good health, and to connect. Taoists believe a man can absorb life energy (known as *chi*) from a woman by having sex with her. Because they believe women have a much bigger supply of this energy than men, it is apparently believed that woman can spare plenty of this life energy without any ill effects. Taoists believe that this life energy can help cure or alleviate a variety of health problems, such as high cholesterol and hormone imbalances.

Ejaculation Control

Under Taoism, seminal fluid is considered a precious life force, so men are encouraged not to "waste" it through unnecessary ejaculation. In fact, for a man in the ancient Tao community, having sex with numerous women in a short period of time without ejaculating at all was considered a feat worthy of much admiration.

So Taoists practice several techniques to help men learn to control (and avoid) ejaculation. One of these involves the perineum, the area of a man between the scrotum and the anus. By applying pressure to this spot immediately before orgasm, it is said that you can block the release of seminal fluid through the urethra when the man climaxes. However, some modern experts criticize this practice, saying it can possibly lead to damage of the perineum and bladder problems (from forcing the semen back up toward the bladder). In addition, critics say, there is no guarantee that this technique can really prevent a man from ejaculating.

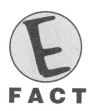

FACT

The area between a man's anus and scrotum (technically known as the *perineum*) has been dubbed "the Million Dollar Point" by Stephen Chang, author of *The Tao of Sexology,* and is now commonly referred to by that term.

Because some men find it physically uncomfortable to reach the brink of orgasm without ejaculation, Taoists also devised exercises designed to divert the blood flow away from the genitals in order to relieve the pressure and swelling in that area. One of these techniques reportedly involved doing a headstand to help the blood flow back toward the stomach and upper body!

Kama Sutra and Tantra

The Kama Sutra is the first written work to focus on the art of lovemaking. To this day, it remains the most well known sex book. Although originally passed down by way of verbal traditions, the book was written by Vatsyayana around A.D. 350. An Englishman named Sir Richard Burton produced the first English language translation in the 1800s. The Kama Sutra was never designed to be a bestseller. It was originally intended just for upper-income men. However, although generally only young men studied it formally with a teacher, young women were taught its lessons as well—they got their instruction from older, married female relatives for instance.

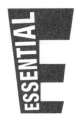

Sir Richard Burton was a famous British scholar, linguist, and explorer. He is not to be confused with the actor of the same name, who lived in the twentieth century and became as famous for his love life (he was married and divorced from Elizabeth Taylor twice) as for his movie credits.

Many people make the mistake of confusing the Kama Sutra with a Tantric how-to sex guide. This would be incorrect. But somewhere along the line, the two did start to become more closely intertwined, perhaps because at quick glance they both fall under the general heading of spiritual approaches to sensual pleasure. However, many of the positions featured in the Kama Sutra have been adapted to fit in with Tantric techniques. "Tantra and the Kama Sutra have a number of things in common," says Al Link, a longtime teacher of Tantra and author of several books on the subject.

In both of them, sexuality is only a small part of the teaching and practices. For example only approximately 50 out of 1250 verses of the Kama Sutra deal with sexual intercourse positions, and in most Tantric practices, sexuality is only introduced very late in the disciple's learning, if at all. Secondly, both Tantra and the Kama Sutra emphasize certain disciplined sexual practices, for example men delaying ejaculation so the lovemaking can be extended for a much longer period of time, or the importance of making sure the female is fully sexually satisfied. Perhaps the major difference between them, is that Tantra is primarily a spiritual practice with a view to the ultimate liberation in enlightenment, while the Kama Sutra is primarily a secular manual of techniques for enhancing relationship and sexuality.

Nineteenth- and Twentieth-Century Revival

Tantra has enjoyed a revival in the West recently. This is perhaps due at least in part to more modern views and attitudes with regard to both sex and spirituality. With the prevalence of "New Age" thinking today, people are more receptive to learning about Tantra and not so likely to be bothered or frightened by its rumored connections to magic or witchcraft.

Tantra was first introduced to Western people in the 1800s by European scholars and people from India and nearby regions. Gradually, the teachings started to spread across the West and Tantra began to develop a growing following.

Alice Bunker Stockham

Interestingly, one of the first people to help bring Tantra to the United States was a woman. Alice Bunker Stockham, a Chicago gynecologist, traveled to India in the nineteenth century because she wanted to learn the secrets of Tantra. As a Christian, Stockham was not interested in learning a new religion. She was, however, eager to learn about the sexual aspects of Tantra. Stockham was definitely considered a rebel in her day. She spoke openly about the benefits of masturbation, discussed birth control options, and was a big believer in women's rights.

Late 1900s

Tantra really started to catch on in the United States during the sexually adventurous '60s and '70s, when the country was experiencing a sexual revolution. The Tantric philosophy meshed well with the whole "free love" spirit of the times. And thanks to major developments like the arrival of the birth control pill and books about sex and sexual pleasure, people were becoming increasingly more open to learning new things about sex. Meanwhile, in other parts of the world, there were also important developments related to Tantra. Toward the end of the twentieth century, an increasing number of Tibetan monks and other exiles began fleeing the oppressive control of the Chinese Communist leadership. Most of these refugees went on to establish Buddhist groups in northern India, where they continue to practice Tantra today. In fact, they are considered to be the "guardians" of Tantra, preserving its traditions and ensuring that it is practiced in its original forms.

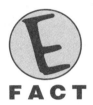

FACT

The Tantric Order in America was founded in 1905. A man named Peter Coon, who was born in Iowa but later changed his name to the more Continental-sounding Pierre Arnold Bernard, is credited with starting the group, which was the first organized Tantric movement in the United States. Bernard would also become known as "Shastri" or "Oom."

Important Figures in Tantric History

There have been many scholars and proponents of Tantra in the Western world. Some of the more pivotal people in the Western movement include:

Sir John Woodroffe

Considered by some to be the founding father of Western Tantric study, Woodroffe was the first Western scholar to seriously look at Tantra. He wrote about the Tantra—under the pseudonym Arthur Avalon—as an ethical philosophy and defended it against its critics. His most famous work is *The Serpent Power: The Secrets of Tantric and Shaktic Yoga.*

Charles Muir

Among the forefathers of the current modern Tantric movement is Charles Muir, who calls himself "the grandfather of the modern Tantra movement in the United States." He created the "Tantra: The Art of Conscious Loving" format of Tantric instruction (based on a book of the same name, which he cowrote with his wife) in 1980 and also developed the art of "sacred spot massage" around the same time.

Margot Anand

Charles Muir may consider himself modern Tantra's grandpa, but Margot Anand has frequently been called the "mother of the modern Tantra movement." Anand, author of many sex books including *The Art of Sexual Ecstasy*, is a highly regarded Tantra teacher and founder of SkyDancing Tantra, a broad group of philosophies and beliefs initially taught by Anand personally and now shared with people worldwide via her Skydancing Institute, books, DVDs, and online resources. She spent many years studying under some of the world's most revered gurus of Buddhist and Hindu Tantra.

Deepak Chopra

Deepak Chopra, author of numerous books, is one of the most well known healers, spiritual leaders, and medical advisors in the United States (and perhaps the world). He is mainly associated with New Age concepts of self-awareness, alternative medicine, and the mind-body connection. Given that, it doesn't seem so surprising that he is also a vocal supporter of Tantric philosophies. He has recommended Tantra as a good way to explore and realize your relationship with nature and the universe.

Tantric Symbols

Symbolism is very important in the Tantric world (as are statues depicting Tantric rituals). There are several symbols (and objects with symbolic meaning) in particular that are seen as having ultimate importance for Tantric followers:

- **Yantras:** A geometrical drawing or configuration, a yantra is considered to have a sacred meaning because its pattern represents a deity.
- **Kapala:** Used as a bowl to contain food or liquids to be offered in a symbolic sacrifice, the kapala is a skull cup. In ancient times, the kapala was actually made from a real human skull. Eventually,

though, it became more common for it to be a cup that was simply fashioned to look like a skull.

- **Mala:** A string of prayer beads, similar in appearance to those used by people of the Christian faith, a typical Tibetan mala would have a minimum of 108 beads. A Tibetan Tantric would often clutch the mala while meditating or reciting his mantras.

- **Vajra:** One of the primary Tantric symbols, the vajra is generally believed to be a combination of a scepter and some kind of weapon. It represents the quality of being strong and indestructible.

- **Bells:** The bell is used in many Tantric rituals as a sound effect. The bell and vajra are often used together, one being held in each hand. In this case, the vajra represents the male form and qualities like strength, while the bell represents females and wisdom. While the vajra and bell both have overall significance as a whole, each component of these symbols also has individual meaning. For example, the vajra's sixteen lotus petals represent the sixteen modes of emptiness in Buddhist beliefs.

- **Swords:** Swords are very common in Tantric symbolism. They represent the ability and strength to cut through negative things like resistance, obstacles, or ignorance.

- **Khatvanga:** A ceremonial Tantric staff, the khatvanga is also sometimes depicted as a magic wand; it symbolizes magic powers or enlightenment.

- **Bumpa:** This is a vase used in traditional Tantric rituals such as initiation ceremonies and healing rites.

- **Tantric Gestures:** Specific gestures hold great symbolic meaning in the practice of Tantra. These ritual hand gestures are called *mudras*, and involve positioning the hands in specific ways that represent things of important sacred meaning.

- **Mandala:** A sacred circle in which the universe, a palace, or some other type of paradise is depicted, a mandala is frequently embellished with jewels or precious metals. Or, mandalas can be made from grains of sand, formed into intricate designs, in a very time-consuming process. Tantrics would often focus on a mandala in order to concentrate during meditation.

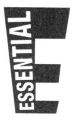

To learn more about important Tantric symbols and the history behind them, check out *The Encyclopedia of Tibetan Symbols and Motifs*, by Robert Beer. The author—a British artist who specializes in Tibetan works—does a great job of illustrating various Tibetan and Tantric symbols in categories like nature, animals, and weapons.

Tantric Terms

Tantra has a unique traditional jargon—you might call it a "language of love." You will learn quite a few of these terms throughout this book (and in the glossary) but here are some basics that might be helpful before you go any further:

- **Yoni:** literal translation is "sacred space," used to refer to the vagina
- **Lingam:** literal translation is "wand of light," refers to the penis
- **Polishing the Pearl:** oral sex on a woman
- **Playing the Flute:** oral sex on a man
- **Jewels:** genitals
- **Sexual union:** intercourse
- **Kundalini:** spiritual energy or life force energy
- **Devamani:** testicles

Chapter 3

The Spiritual Side of Tantra

Many westerners are intrigued by Tantra because of its sexual aspects. They simply want a way to make their sex lives more exciting. But there is so much more to Tantra than that. The real crux of Tantra—the critical issue of utmost importance to dedicated Tantrics—is the spiritual aspect. Spirituality is seen as the key to achieving balance and unity with other people and the world. Tantrics believe that by nurturing your spirit, you allow everything else to fall into place in a positive way.

Why Spirit Is Important in Tantra

The basic philosophy of Tantra boils down to the importance of your spirit. Tantrics believe that each of us embody the sacred spirit. According to Tantric teachings, everything you do in life should be about honoring and nourishing this divine spirit. Your spirit should have a positive energy and a strong connection with the world around you. This should be your primary goal, one you should never forget. It is important to nurture your spirit and allow it to grow and flourish happily. If your spirit is in a positive place, your physical and mental well-being will follow.

This extends to the issue of sex. When you use Tantric teachings to treat your spirit to a healthy, happy, and exciting sex life, you attain ultimate bliss. In other words, once your spirit is in sync, the good sex will follow.

Spirituality Versus Religion

Many people often confuse spirituality and religion. There is much debate surrounding the difference between the two terms. However, the important thing is to recognize that the two are not interchangeable and can mean two vastly different things to some people.

The spiritual may be seen as what is born from the inside. It is what guides us in our daily lives, the emotion behind the practice. Spirituality is the essence of our soul, and what is in our innermost nature.

By contrast, religion may be seen as the practice itself, the rituals and theory guiding it all. The practice, for some, may be empty movements void of feeling, or spirit. You probably know people who claim to be highly religious but in reality are just very good at going through all of the formal motions. For others, the religious practice may be the portal for the spiritual—what increases it and expresses it.

How Tantra Fits In

Tantra is not a religion at all, but an ancient set of spiritual beliefs. Tantra has never become an actual religion, and it was never intended to be one—partly because by its very nature it is not conducive to the set of structured guidelines and formats associated with most religions. With Tantra, there are no commandments or strict rules to follow. You are not required to maintain a rigid prayer schedule or attend services at designated times. You are not excommunicated or ostracized if you do not adhere to strict rules. Each Tantric practitioner dictates his or her own path based on what's right for that individual. This is how it has always been. Tantra was originally passed from guru to student, and each guru had his own unique approach to the Tantra beliefs.

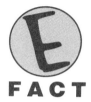

Not only is Tantra not a religion, but in some ways it actually started out as an anti-religion. Early Tantrics embraced the beliefs as a welcome change from the strict and repressive religions of that time, which had a very elitist attitude, as only a select group of high-class people were deemed worthy of religious teachings.

Thoughts from a Tantra Teacher

Somraj Pokras, founder of Tantra at Tahoe, has this to say about Tantra and religions:

> *Religions are often based on dogmatic beliefs and can sometimes impose attitudes and require rituals from members regardless of the individual impact. Tantra is based on an individual's experience as the central focus of practice. Further, Tantra is based on opening one's kundalini energy channels, so it's all about practicing to feel the subtle energy awaken and grow. What you think, what you believe, what you talk about is secondary in Tantra.*

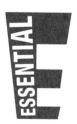

The most obvious way that Tantra differs from most religions involves sex. Most modern religions view sex as something to be shared between husband and wife, and even then usually for the purpose of procreation. In fact, many people get the impression from religious advisors that sex is something bad or dirty. By contrast, Tantrics believe sex is a sacred gift.

Tantra's Role in Religion Today

Today, most Tantrics view Tantra as something that complements—rather than replaces—whatever religion the person is currently observing. Tantrics come from all walks of life and just about every religion imaginable. The key is to successfully blend the Tantra philosophies with those of your religious beliefs.

Here are some more thoughts from Somraj Pokras about Tantra and religion.

> *Today Tantrics revere Shiva as the pure embodiment of the masculine force culminating in cosmic consciousness, and Shakti as the feminine principle embodying pure creative energy. This isn't worship of supreme beings as in most organized religions. Rather, it is Tantra's way of honoring the forces of nature that exist within each of us. We simply use Shiva and Shakti as convenient symbols to focus the growth of our own divine qualities.*

Making a Connection Is Crucial

In order to begin Tantric practice with your partner, you must make a connection. This is crucial to the process of spiritual awakening.

The purpose of Tantric sex is to build the connection between you and your partner, thereby breaking down boundaries and forming a strong, intimate bond. In this way, you overcome fears, insecurities, get in touch with your own body, and become more aware of your partner's body and soul.

Many women (and even a considerable number of men) do not easily reach orgasm. This is often due to emotional and psychological obstacles, as opposed to physical problems. Making that connection with one's partner is essential to heightening orgasmic potential. We get so caught up in the stress of everyday life, that even sex becomes monotonous. By slowing down and taking the time to really notice and appreciate each other, we increase our sexual awareness and open the doors to complete satisfaction and full intimacy.

Building the Connection

There are various ways you can increase this intimate connection before beginning to make love. You take the first step by creating a sacred environment, a sanctuary for you and your lover. By taking the time to gaze at one another before sex, you are forging that sacred bond. Eye gazing is basic to Tantric practices. That alone can lead you to mind-altering bliss. Massages, both sensual and sexual, are also excellent ways to make that initial connection.

The yoga asanas (poses or postures) and the rituals presented in this book are all ways to establish the necessary connection with your partner. After all, you are traveling this holy path together. You are learning and exploring together. You must learn to open up to your partner and become vulnerable. You are each other's guide, each other's guru.

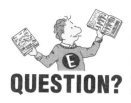

QUESTION?

What are some ways to build a connection?
There are many ways that you can establish a connection with your partner on a daily basis. Next time you touch your partner, focus on the sensations. Do it deliberately and for just a moment, and abandon yourself to the sensation. Also try to say "yes" more often to your loved one's requests, both sexually and otherwise. You may be surprised at the results.

Awaken the Passion

When couples have been together for a significant amount of time, they have a tendency to fall into a routine and forget about that deep intimacy and romance they shared at the beginning. Tantric practices reconnect the couple, reawaken that lustful passion and redirect it. It is no longer passion for the sake of satisfaction. It is a deep passion planted in fertile soil—that is, a love and understanding that is cultivated and cared for and now used to achieve spiritual bliss together.

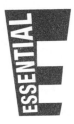

Communication is key to forming a connection. This means that honesty and vulnerability are welcome in the bedroom. You and your partner need the space to say what you feel, want, and need both emotionally and physically. If this is done with compassion and tenderness, your relationship will grow and flourish.

When people enter into a new relationship and are in that "honeymoon" stage, they are often carried away by the excitement of lustful longing and a new adventure. Tantric practices also help to harness this energy. Rather than starting out strong and quickly burning out, Tantra regulates it, sets a pace, and directs it into disciplined ecstasy. This gives the couple the bases, trust, and compassion that they need not only to have great sex, but also to continue having it into the future.

Consciousness and Tantra

Consciousness is a term you hear a lot in relation to Tantra. Tantrics believe that human beings are just miniature representations of the universe, and that therefore if you access your spirits by way of your senses through consciousness of yoga, meditation, and sacred love, you find the key that will unlock the secrets of godly wisdom. As a result, you will become a god or goddess. In other words, gods and goddesses are simply people who have recognized the cosmic potential within themselves and attained their fullest potential level of consciousness.

Thoughts on Consciousness from an Expert

Longtime Tantra teacher Al Link elaborates on the concept of consciousness:

> *Everything is consciousness. Consciousness is what we come out of and what we go back into. If we are diligent and determined, we can come to this realization while we are in the seemingly separate space of a body. We can become aware, not just*

with our minds, but with all aspects of our being, that everything is indeed one. Unlike many spiritual practices that suggest we must deny or escape the body to come to such an awareness, Tantra teaches that the body is a gateway through to awakening. Our desires are fuel for the fire of awareness. Our senses are the doorways through to perception. By being fully present—awake, alive, focused—in our bodies, we can tune in to the subtle vibration at the core of all life and know we are everything and everything is us.

Shiva and Shakti and Their Role in Consciousness

Tantra teaches us that the universe is consciousness. This consciousness is both masculine and feminine. Shiva, the masculine force, is solid and unchanging. It is possibility and pure potential. Shakti, the feminine force, is always changing. It is dynamic and creative. From her, all else springs forth.

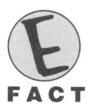

FACT

Ancient Tantrics viewed Shiva as a powerful force in the universe (modern Tantrics still maintain this view). Shiva was often associated with death, or the ending of life's energy. Shatki was Shiva's consort, and provided feminine balance to the equation.

This is where the energy of kundalini comes in. The feminine force that is Shakti is called kundalini in the human body. Kundalini resides at the base of the spinal cord. It can be awakened through kundalini yoga asanas, meditations, and rituals. Once kundalini is awakened, we are provided with a life force beyond everyday understanding. It allows us to fully experience our spiritual as well as worldly lives, as the line separating the two becomes almost nonexistent.

Tantra tries to carry us beyond the dualities of masculine and feminine. By awakening our consciousness to ourselves, we awake our consciousness to the universe. We move beyond the dualities imposed by human minds. We move beyond the ego and for a moment, we experience pure bliss.

Subconsciousness and Superconsciousness

While we are on the subject of consciousness, it is fitting to discuss two other states of consciousness: the subconscious and the superconscious. You are probably familiar with the idea of subconscious actions. This is when we do something almost automatically, without really even thinking about it or perhaps without even knowing why we are acting this way. Subconscious actions are often based on instinct or intuition, rather than a long thought-out logical process. Our subconscious is also like our mind's safety-deposit box. This is where it stores memories, thoughts, and experiences—including those that we may not want to remember, and which we may in fact believe we have forgotten.

Then there is the idea of superconsciousness. As you can probably guess from the name, this is when you reach the ultimate level of consciousness—complete mental and spiritual clarity. This is a state of ultimate bliss, a place many Tantrics aspire to reach someday.

Osho and Superconsciousness

Osho was a well-known and controversial Indian spiritual guide and teacher of the twentieth century. He earned a reputation (and not necessarily a good one) as a sex guru after giving some speeches in the 1960s that dealt with sexual content that some conservative critics found scandalous. Some of his speeches served as the basis for a book called *From Sex to Superconsciousness*. In this book, Osho discusses the three stages of sex—physical, psychological, and spiritual—and offers advice on channeling this raw energy into the realization of ultimate consciousness.

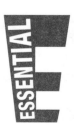

One of Osho's most well known quotes is from *Philosophia Perennis* and goes like this: "If you have not explored your body, you will not be able to explore the soul. The methodology of exploration is the same, but begin with the body because it is the visible part of your soul. Start with the visible and then slowly move toward the invisible."

Osho believed that when we repress our basic nature, sex takes root in the unconscious, creating an unnatural obsession. According to Osho, this psychological state has produced a mental sickness and widespread, unhealthy obsession within society today. Therefore, you might say that he considered sexual exploration and indulging your personal needs as a valuable contribution that you make to society and the world in general.

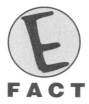

FACT

Some Tantrics believe that by mastering a state of consciousness a person can achieve amazing and unbelievable things—even traveling through time and space. They believe that as someone reaches the ultimate state of superconsciousness, he or she may be able to visit past lifetimes.

Important Tantric Teachings

When it comes to Tantra, spirituality, and consciousness, there are some important things to keep in mind:

- Sex is just one of the vehicles that can carry us to the state of pure bliss. Just as we contain the same elements as the universe, each one of us is comprised of opposing types of characteristics: masculine and feminine, good and bad, dark and light. Tantra teaches us to let go of preconceived ideas and reach a state of spiritual awakening. This, then, is true consciousness, breaking free from polarities. As you perfect the Tantric art and cultivate your sensibilities, you will expand into higher and higher dimensions of consciousness.

- Tantra also teaches us that we do not belong to anyone or anything. By the same token, nothing belongs to us, either. We are all a small part of the cosmic consciousness. What exists without also exists within. In other words, we are all miniatures of the universe.

- In our personal relationships, we often enter into games of power and possession. Inevitably, these cause us pain, confusion, and anger and result in all sorts of negative reactions. When we are accustomed to acting in this way, it tends to become a repetitive cycle. Tantra teaches us to move away from those patterns. It is essential to keep in mind that you do not belong to your partner and he or she does not belong to you. You are separate beings who are fortunate enough to be able to intertwine in a state of spiritual bliss. There are no boundaries.

- Tantrics believe that an important way to achieve consciousness is to love and accept yourself for who you are and what you stand for. This consciousness then stimulates your higher spiritual and sexual powers.

- Tantra requires dedication. One must dedicate time for thought and meditation, and time to be with one's partner. In order to tap into our spiritual selves, we must increase awareness, deepen our breathing, listen more carefully, and practice with our partner. Once you begin the Tantric path and begin to feel the effects it has on your life, you will not want to go back. As you grow in spiritual awareness, you will be that much closer to knowing your partner and yourself, ultimately, and pure bliss.

Chapter 4

Understanding the Orgasm

Ah, the all-important orgasm. It is known by a variety of nicknames: the Big O, the point of no return, climax, cumming, and even "the money shot." Whatever you call it, orgasm is an important part of the sexual experience. To many people, it is considered the *most* important, the grand finale—a way to wrap up the sexual encounter and "bring it on home." But the orgasm is also one of the most misunderstood aspects of the whole sexual experience.

Introduction to Orgasms

As most people probably already know, an orgasm is a sexual climax. The word *orgasm* is based on a Greek term meaning "to swell." In Tantra, orgasm is seen as a divine experience. But in following the Tantric tradition of slow and leisurely lovemaking, the goal is generally to prolong orgasm as long as possible.

The Traditional View

In traditional Tantra, orgasm wasn't viewed with the obsession that it is by many people today. In fact, orgasm was often discouraged—if not outright prohibited—because it was seen as a waste of vital energy forces. Orgasm was something that was not to be done haphazardly or taken lightly. A couple who engaged in a fulfilling, spiritually rewarding lovemaking session certainly would not have been considered a failure simply because one or both partners did not achieve orgasm.

The Modern Cultural View

On the other hand, the modern sexual viewpoint is to place the utmost importance on orgasm. It is often all some people seem to focus on, almost to the point of obsession. Frankly, there's a lot of pressure to have one (mainly for women) and in some cases this can actually detract from the pleasure of the experience—thus, the popularity of "faking it." But, as everyone can probably agree, faking it is no solution, and it really does not end up benefiting anyone.

The Four Stages of Sexual Response

In order to better understand orgasms, it is helpful to evaluate their place in the grand scheme of things, sexually speaking. Sex research pioneers Masters and Johnson established four phases of human sexual response: excitement, plateau, orgasm, and resolution. It will probably be enlightening for you to examine each phase in greater detail.

Excitement Stage

The very first stage of human sexual response is the excitement stage. This is the stage that is least likely to be obvious, as it can (and often does) occur before any apparent stimulation or contact has taken place. The excitement or arousal stage often begins immediately upon any kind of romantic physical contact, including kissing. It can also occur as a result of visual stimulation, such as viewing X-rated movies, adult magazines, or anything else the person finds arousing. At this point, we as rational humans know in our minds that sexual activity is not necessarily a foregone conclusion, but the body does not, so it instinctively starts making preparations for the sex it believes will soon happen. The arousal period is physically noticeable by some clear-cut signs. The first is enlargement and engorgement of the genital areas and other parts of the body. This occurs in both men and women. With men, it is pretty blatant—the penis becomes hard, erect, and larger. With women, they experience vaginal engorgement as well as hardening/enlargement of areas of the breast. Both women and men may experience a redness or flushing of the skin, especially on their face and chest.

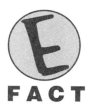

FACT

Despite being known as one of the biggest female sex symbols of recent times—and being linked to a long list of high-profile men—Marilyn Monroe reportedly confessed to a friend that she had never had an orgasm.

Plateau Stage

When excitement progresses, the body reaches the plateau stage of sexual response. At this point, the physical signs increase—the breasts, penis, and vaginal areas become more enlarged and engorged, breathing gets even more rapid and sweating may occur. At this point, men may excrete what is commonly referred to as preseminal fluid. If it did not already happen during the excitement stage, women generally start to experience vaginal lubrication during this stage. When women are in the plateau stage, their clitoris also becomes enlarged. If the process is halted at this point, both men and women may experience some discomfort but—contrary to the claims of some teenage boys—there is no evidence that this can cause any permanent harm.

Orgasm Stage

The orgasm is the most obvious and impressive stage of human sexual response. This is the period where a lot of things happen in rapid succession in a very short period of time.

There are the obvious physical events, such as the intense muscle contractions, the excretions of fluids, and the rapid breathing. There are also the internal events like the rush of endorphins and other chemicals in the brain and the emotional effects. During orgasm, many people also experience involuntary actions such as moaning, yelling, etc.

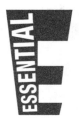

During orgasm, the heart beats an average of 140 times per minute. By contrast, a typical resting heart rate is about 70 beats per minute for a man and 75 beats per minute for a woman. But don't worry: There is no real danger of overstressing your heart. After all, the average orgasm only lasts a fleeting three to eight seconds.

Resolution Stage

The resolution stage is what many people are most likely to call the "recovery stage." This is where the body (and mind) starts to return to a normal state and recover from the stress and excitement of sexual activity. Many people feel tired at this stage, partly due to the physical exertion of sex and partly due to the chemical changes occurring in their brain. Also, it is common for people—especially women—to have strong emotional reactions during this phase, sometimes to the point of crying.

Orgasm Basics

Obviously, there are some fundamental differences between orgasms in men and women, just based on anatomical design alone. But there are many universal orgasm basics that apply to everyone. During actual orgasm, the main physical sign is muscle contractions. There will often be a marked increase in heart rate and blood pressure.

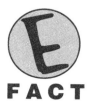

FACT

Karezza is a term used for the technique of learning to control the orgasm response using various techniques including breathing routines and finger pressure. It is sometimes also used as a general term for Tantric-style sacred sex. The term was coined by Alice Bunker Stockham, a doctor and author who is considered a female pioneer in Tantra.

Biological Response

Essentially, there are three anatomical systems involved in the biological response to arousal and orgasm. First, there is the muscular element, which is the most noticeable due to the telltale muscle contractions associated with orgasm. There is also the circulatory element involved when blood rushes to the genital area, breasts, and other aroused parts of the body. Lastly, the neurological system is also involved, because arousal causes a rush of hormones and other chemicals to flood the brain. It is actually somewhat shocking to realize all of the work the body must do in order to have an orgasm, isn't it?

Tantric Orgasms

Tantric teachings address two different types of orgasms: the physical variety and the spiritual one. This second type of orgasm is also referred to as a "heart orgasm" or "energy orgasm." Ideally, a person achieves one ultimate orgasm that combines both physical and spiritual bliss, leading to an amazingly powerful state of consciousness. Tantrics believe it is only then that you can use lovemaking as a way to transcend into a higher spiritual place.

Multiple Orgasms

Multiple orgasms are a series of orgasms that occur (usually in rapid succession) during a single sexual encounter. Many women can achieve multiple orgasms with just a very brief "recovery period" in between, or none at all. Other women need to recharge a bit after each orgasm before attempting to achieve another.

While multiple orgasms are most commonly associated with women, men can experience this phenomenon as well. It is generally easier for younger men to achieve multiple orgasms. Although men can have multiple orgasms, they can usually only ejaculate once during a single sexual session.

Dry Orgasms

A popular Tantric technique involves "dry orgasms," or orgasms without ejaculation. This is designed to allow people to benefit from the "release" of an orgasm without the "grand finale" aspect that is often connected with ejaculation.

Mastering the Technique

A lot of men who achieve multiple orgasms on a regular basis do so after mastering the technique of having dry orgasms, usually through a lot of trial and error. However, some men find dry orgasms to be uncomfortable or even painful. Plus, it is not an easy task to master, often taking lots of practice. Basically, it requires tightly contracting pubococcygeus muscles (the same ones used to stop the flow of urine when going to the bathroom) at the simultaneous moment of orgasm. This requires a lot of self-control and awareness on the part of the man, which is a tall order considering many men have trouble focusing when they are about to climax.

Temporarily Drying Up the Well

If a man has several orgasms in a very short period of time, he will begin to have dry orgasms (whether he wants to or not) because he has basically used up all of his available supply of seminal fluid and caused his ejaculate to "dry up." This lasts only a short time, however, because the body can re-stock seminal fluid very quickly. Normally, the man's seminal reservoir is well stocked again within a few hours.

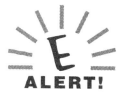

ALERT!

There is a new product called the Aneros Prostate Massager that is designed to help men achieve powerful, dry, full-body orgasms in rapid succession. According to men who have tried this product, it results in an entirely different (yet extremely pleasurable) climax than a "normal" orgasm. You can learn more about this product at ✍ *www.aneros.com*.

The term *dry orgasm* is also sometimes used to mean an orgasm of the mind—a mental orgasm, if you will, where no ejaculation is attempted or desired.

Orgasm Facts and Fallacies

From the time we are in junior high school (or perhaps earlier) we are bombarded with all kinds of rumors, myths, old wives' tales, and just flat-out lies involving sex and, more specifically, orgasms. Let's try to sort out fact from fiction when it comes to this important topic.

Orgasm Facts

Here are some interesting facts related to orgasms:

- An orgasm is a totally normal, natural process. In fact, researches have discovered that infants experience involuntary orgasms within the first few weeks of life. And, of course, some people have experienced orgasms in their sleep.
- Most people who claim they "can't" have an orgasm are actually physically capable of experiencing an orgasm—they simply do not know how. This is especially common among women.

- Both men and women are most likely to experience their first orgasm through masturbation.
- Involuntary orgasms during sleep (known as "wet dreams") can happen to both genders, although this tends to be more common in men.
- In a survey conducted by ABC News, almost half the female respondents said they have faked an orgasm. By contrast, only 11 percent of men said they had faked it. In the same survey, 75 percent of sexually active men said they "always" have an orgasm, while only 30 percent of women said the same.

Orgasm Fallacies

There are lots of myths, misconceptions, and outright lies surrounding orgasms. One of the most prevalent? Many people believe orgasm and ejaculation are synonymous and interchangeable. Tantra views these as two distinctly different and separate occurrences.

There is also the idea that female ejaculation is a myth. Many people are surprised to learn that female ejaculation does indeed exist. Even more surprising, it is something that apparently can be taught and learned. This is evidenced by the numerous books and videos available on the topic.

Male Orgasm Myths

A lot of commonly believed myths surround the male orgasm. First, many people believe men are not capable of experiencing multiple orgasms. In fact, Tantra teaches some techniques that are designed to help men experience more than one orgasm during a single session.

There is also the belief that prolonging orgasm is painful (physically and mentally) for the man, and prolonging orgasm is often seen as something negative, a type of punishment or something the man tolerates just for the woman's sake. However, Tantra teaches the importance and benefits of prolonging orgasm, and how it can in fact be *more* pleasurable.

Orgasms in Men

When people think of male orgasm, their first (and often only) thought is immediately of ejaculation. Ejaculation is a process in which the prostate contracts (along with muscles at the base of the penis) to help push seminal fluid through the urethra and out of the body. And indeed, the dual events of orgasm and ejaculation do often go hand-in-hand.

Men generally only have one type of orgasm—that resulting from direct stimulation of the penis. A smaller percentage of men can achieve orgasm via stimulation of the prostate gland, which usually occurs by way of anal stimulation. However, a lot of men are uncomfortable about anything related to anal stimulation at all, and find just the thought of this to be a complete turnoff.

Orgasms in Women

Fortunately for women, they are able to benefit from a much greater variety of orgasms than men.

Vaginal Orgasm

Some women claim not to have vaginal orgasms, and it is very possible they are telling the truth. Indeed, this type of orgasm can be tricky to achieve. For one thing, the vagina is not exactly optimally designed for maximum orgasmic potential—most of the sensations are felt in the first (outer) third of the vagina. (However, experts and researchers such as Barbara Keesling have discussed the pleasure potential of the "cul-de-sac"—an area at the back of the vaginal canal, just behind where the cervix enters the vagina. Women can experience very intense orgasms with stimulation here. Some refer to this as "the X-spot."). In actuality, when most people talk about a vaginal orgasm, they are more specifically referring to a G-Spot orgasm.

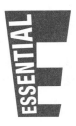

ESSENTIAL

In her well-known book *The Art of Sexual Ecstasy*, Margo Anand describes over a dozen different types of orgasms, including: the penile and prostatic orgasms in men, the anal orgasm in both sexes, and local orgasms of the breast, throat, and lower spine. She also differentiates between the explosive orgasm of outward release and the implosive orgasm of inward expansion.

G-Spot Orgasm

For something so small, the G-spot has certainly managed to get lots of attention—and stir up more than its share of controversy. Some people don't believe it exists at all, while others swear by its ability to produce unparalleled pleasure.

The G-Spot is a small area within the upper wall of the vagina, about one to two inches from the opening. Some women have the ability to reach orgasm through direct stimulation of the G-Spot or gentle massage of the area. When the G-Spot is stimulated, the woman will often feel as if she has the urge to urinate. And, in fact, during a G-Spot orgasm, many women will mistakenly believe they have accidentally urinated. This is because a G-Spot orgasm is notable because it is usually accompanied by a lot of fluid. This is generally referred to as "female ejaculation."

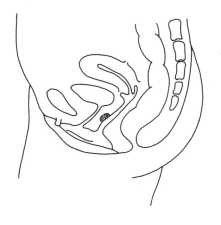

◀ Figure 4-1 Location of the G-Spot

Men, do not despair if you have trouble finding your partner's G-spot. Many women cannot even find their own G-spot easily, so it is not surprising that it would be a challenge for a man to locate this elusive yet magical place.

Clitoral Orgasm

The clitoral orgasm is generally viewed as the easiest type of orgasm for a woman to achieve. Some women also deem it the most pleasurable, but other women who experience G-spot orgasm, X-spot, or whole-body orgasm may disagree with that. In fact, many women are unable to achieve orgasm unless the clitoris is stimulated, even if this occurs only indirectly by way of friction from intercourse. However, this is often because, with most sexual encounters, women don't get enough time to awaken their vaginas and the sensitive spots internally to experience orgasm through stimulation of them. If lovemaking was extended long enough to really, really arouse a woman before penetration, it is a safe bet that lots more women would be experiencing more than clitoral orgasm.

This is reflected by women's habits when it comes to self-pleasure. When masturbating, the majority of women focus on clitoral stimulation and bring themselves to orgasm solely in this way, since they have learned that this is often the quickest and most efficient route to orgasm.

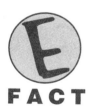

FACT

The word *clitoris* is based on a Greek word meaning "little hill." Most people don't realize that the clitoris is much bigger than it seems—it actually extends up into the body for several inches. The clitoris is also the only genital organ designed purely for pleasure—meaning, it serves no role in the reproductive process at all.

Are Female Orgasms "Necessary"?

Throughout history, the orgasms of men were viewed with more respect because they were considered to have a functional and vital purpose— the transfer of sperm in order to procreate. By contrast, female orgasms were seen as a "luxury," an indulgence purely for pleasure. It was believed that they served no biological purpose and therefore were largely considered unnecessary. Not everyone shared that view, though. In the fourth century B.C., Hippocrates stated his belief that in order for a woman to become pregnant, she must achieve orgasm. However, his peer Aristotle disputed this, and as a result female pleasure continued to be dismissed as unimportant.

But recently this debate has come to life again, as researchers and other notable figures are again arguing about whether the female orgasm serves any functional and essential purpose. Some experts believe female orgasm helps create a "suction" effect that aids the sperm in reaching the uterus, thus making pregnancy more likely.

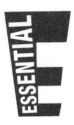

In his 1953 book *Sexual Behavior in the Human Female*, Dr. Alfred A. Kinsey found that 39 to 47 percent of women reported that they always, or almost always, had orgasm during intercourse.

But others are unconvinced that the female orgasm is necessary, biologically speaking. In a book called *The Case of the Female Orgasm: Bias in the Science of Evolution*, published in 2005, Dr. Elisabeth A. Lloyd, a professor of biology at Indiana University, examines twenty leading theories about the evolutionary purpose of female orgasm. She finds flaws with all of them, and in the end reaches the conclusion that female orgasms serve no evolutionary function at all.

Full-Body Orgasm

Tantra philosophy stresses the importance of a full-body orgasm. This is a combination of the physical orgasm and the "heart orgasm." As its name implies, the full-body orgasm involves the entire anatomy—all of the senses, plus the mind. It is said to be a more extended form of orgasm, often involving several peaks and valleys before the final climax. Many Tantric gurus believe a person could have orgasms that focused on areas of the body outside the genital region—such as the breasts, throat, or spine—when those areas reached peak stimulation levels.

Simultaneous Orgasms

A lot of couples strive to have simultaneous orgasms—meaning, when both partners climax at the same time (sometimes also called matching orgasms). While this is great when it happens, some people feel it is overrated—and in fact, it can end up having a negative effect because couples can get so preoccupied with one partner trying to "catch up" to the other that the experience falls short. Many couples find it is easier to achieve simultaneous orgasms after they have been together for a while, when they have become familiar with their partner's signs of impending climax and have developed a knack for getting in sync with each other's rhythm. Still, it is advisable not to obsess over pursuing this goal, or you will surely miss out on some potentially great sexual moments.

Enhancing Orgasms

While many people are quite content just to have any kind of orgasm at all, there are ways that even the best orgasm can be improved upon. Let's take a look at some of the ways to enhance your orgasm.

PC Exercises

Strengthening their PC (pubococcygeal) muscles can help women enjoy sex—and as a result, orgasms—much more than before. The PC muscles are those pelvic muscles that you would contract in order to stop the flow of urine. How do you strengthen these muscles? By doing what are known as Kegel exercises. Basically, this involves squeezing those muscles several times in a row on a frequent basis. Tip for women: Try squeezing these muscles while having intercourse. You will basically be making a tight grip around your partner's penis—and will certainly grab his attention, as well.

Allowing Arousal to Subside

Another way of enhancing orgasm is to prolong your climax. As you start nearing that point, pause for a moment, do some deep breathing, and allow your climax to subside a bit. You can repeat this process several times, heightening the anticipation of the moment when you finally do climax. This is sometimes referred to as the stop-start technique.

Sex Toys and Products

These days, enhancing your sex life and/or orgasm seems to be as easy as heading to the mall or sitting in front of your computer and visiting an online adult store. There are lots of adult toys (including many available online) that promise to help enhance your orgasm. Recently, the market has also been flooded with an endless variety of creams, gels, and other products designed to enhance orgasms. With these products, there is no "one size fits all" answer. An enhancement product that one person finds helpful and enjoyable may produce a sensation that someone else finds unpleasant. Especially when it comes to the enhancement creams, you will find a real variety of quality and results. Many of the creams (especially the low-priced ones) seem to be nothing more than a dose of menthol, similar to what moms use to rub on the chests of sick children to open their sinuses. These can produce a tingly sensation when rubbed on the genitals, but in some cases it is more like an unpleasant burning sensation. So try a few products yourself and do your own "bedroom tests."

Benefits of Orgasm

Orgasms are not just enjoyable and emotionally fulfilling; they can also offer benefits to your physical health. Researchers have cited lots of physical benefits resulting from orgasms, including shiny hair, glowing skin, and improved circulation. Even better, having regular orgasms can help your cardiovascular health, boost your immune system, improve your strength and flexibility, and maybe even help with symptoms of menstrual cramps, arthritis, and other medical conditions. In addition, the chemical changes resulting from orgasms can help alleviate symptoms of depression and anxiety.

Chapter 5

Getting Started

The hardest part of tackling anything that is new or unknown is taking that all-important first step. Trying something new, no matter what it is, can be scary. While Tantra's mysterious air and ancient roots can make it seem tough to grasp at first, it most likely will be easier than you think. Plus, this is one educational experience that will really be lots of fun. Not to mention, the Tantric community is well known for being warm and welcoming to "newbies" with a sincere desire to learn.

Are You Really Ready?

Before going any further, it is important to look inside yourself and honestly assess your readiness to explore Tantra. Be totally sincere with yourself about your interest (or lack of it) in pursuing this. You may not be ready for this step at this specific point in your life. Jumping into this experience just because you think it sounds "cool" or trendy, or because you just met a hot new girl and want to impress her with some new tricks in your sexual repertoire may not be the best motivation. So let's explore your readiness to start this road to Tantric enlightenment.

Open Your Mind

Perhaps the most important thing you need in order to start this journey is an open mind. Forget any preconceived notions you may have of Tantra and the people who practice it. Many people have heard various myths and misconceptions involving Tantra and related topics like the Kama Sutra and Taoism. In most cases, these notions are based on false stereotypical images that are completely off the mark. Most people find that Tantra is completely different from what they expected and are pleasantly surprised by what they discover. This very likely could turn out to be true in your case, as well.

Leave Your Preconceived Notions Behind

It is important that you do not walk into this with any prejudices or ulterior motives, or you will be sure to fail. In order to benefit from Tantric teachings, you must approach it with a totally open mind, receptive to new and different ideas and beliefs.

You must be open to exploring ideas that may seem strange or totally foreign to you at first. It is also important that you are not afraid of appearing silly or "different." To many people, some of the techniques encouraged in Tantra—the romantic rituals for example, or the chanting and breathing techniques—may feel awkward, uncomfortable, or even embarrassing at first. Do not give in to these feelings. They will only impede your spiritual awakening. Allowing yourself to be controlled by your inhibitions or fears will make it difficult for you to fully benefit from the wonders of Tantra.

The First Steps

Okay, so you are honestly ready and eager to study Tantra, but don't know where to start? Well, congratulations, you are already on your way. You may not realize it, but just by reading this book, you have taken a great—an important—first step in your quest for Tantric enlightenment. Selecting this book demonstrates that you have a serious desire to learn and the willingness to make an effort—two of the most important characteristics of a successful Tantric-in-training. You are on your way!

Do Some Research

Before diving into any important new experience, you should do some legwork and get as much information as possible. Think about it: These days, many people don't even dare try a new restaurant without first checking online reviews, e-mailing friends asking for the scoop, plotting the location on MapQuest.com to evaluate the drive, etc. Needless to say, you should put at least that much minimal effort into deciding whether to pursue something that just possibly may change your entire outlook on life.

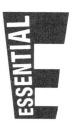

Robin Taylor is a therapist and sexologist who specializes in Tantric topics. Her advice for aspiring Tantrics? "Start reading. The purest of the ideas are all available in print. Classes are good, but many practitioners are still run by ego, or by unhealed stuff of their own."

When you are first exploring the idea of Tantra and sacred sexuality, books are a good starting point. There are many wonderful and thorough books (and e-books) available that can prove very helpful to an aspiring Tantric.

Ironically, modern technology has made it easier than ever to study the ancient art of Tantra. By doing a quick online search, you will find more Tantra-related Web sites than you can count. Many of these sites also allow you to register for classes, workshops, and retreats. Some also have bulletin boards or online groups where you can "meet" and mingle with other, more experienced Tantrics who will probably be happy to share their insights and answer your questions. Ideally, you will connect with a few relatively new Tantrics who can still clearly recall what it was like to be in your position and can offer some valuable support and advice.

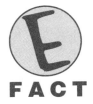

FACT

Many of the top Tantra Web sites sell books, informative CDs, and other materials that can help you learn a lot about Tantra. Even better, these sites often allow you to buy e-books, which you can then download and read instantly. You can often find material specifically geared toward people who are new to Tantra and want to get started.

A lot of people find CDs and videos to be a very convenient way to learn about Tantra. Just the soothing, friendly tone of the teacher's voice can often be a good preview of the meditative benefits you may get from Tantric techniques. Also, it is sometimes reassuring to see "normal-looking" people practicing the techniques (as opposed to the exotic swami-type guru you may be picturing in your mind).

What Are Your Needs?

It is important to spend some time evaluating your needs, considering your reasons for studying Tantra, and clarifying your goals. What do you hope to get out of it? Are there specific benefits you seek, or things you hope to gain? Give particular thought to areas in which you feel your life is lacking something, and ways in which Tantra might be able to help fill those voids.

If you are in a committed relationship, think about whether your partner will share your interests—and if so, how this shared journey can affect you and your partner, individually and as a unit. This is important, as a joint Tantric learning journey can be a wonderful experience, as long as both partners share the same interest.

Do not rush this process. Take your time, and really ponder your main priorities in pursuing Tantra, and what you ideally hope to gain.

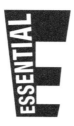

You may want to create an informal Tantra chart to give you a fresh perspective on a situation you are facing. List things you feel are missing or lacking in your life, or things about yourself you would like to improve. Then jot down a few ways you think Tantra may be able to assist in making those plans/goals a reality.

Purpose of Self-Evaluation

There are really no right and wrong answers to these questions. Each person is different, with a unique situation. This self-evaluation is not to determine whether your reasons for studying Tantra are "good" or not. Nobody—especially your fellow Tantrics—will feel like they have the right to judge your motivations. People will have many different reasons for pursuing this knowledge. Your answers are for your knowledge alone and will simply serve as a guideline as to how you should proceed.

This assessment and evaluation process is important because Tantra is such a vast philosophy, covering a broad spectrum of material and ideas. In addition, there are several different varieties of Tantra—mainly the two "branches": traditional (Eastern) Tantra and Neo-Tantra.

If you seek spiritual enlightenment and are open to exploring an entire system of beliefs based on thousands of years of tradition, then the Eastern version of Tantra is probably what you seek. However, this type of Tantra involves abstract ideas and considerable history, so it isn't the kind of thing you can learn overnight.

On the other hand, if you mainly want a way to spice up your sex life or strengthen an intimate bond with your partner, you should focus on studying Neo-Tantra. Remember, your decision is not carved in stone. You will not be "locked in" to one type of Tantra for the rest of your life. Many people start out studying one type of Tantra and later end up studying another approach, either in addition to or in place of their original choice.

Advice from the Experts

Al Link and Pala Copeland are longtime Tantra teachers and authors who have counseled many new aspiring Tantrics. They share this advice for people new to the subject: "Beginners who wish to explore Tantra can learn a great deal from reading even one book or attending one weekend workshop. On the other hand, you can go on learning more for the rest of your life. The most important thing is to get started by experimenting to find which of the many approaches, methods, and techniques appeal to you and feel right when you try them."

Al and Pala offer these suggestions to help you take small steps into the world of Tantra:

- Start paying attention to your body's messages—listen to it, inside and out. Do a body scan, starting at your head or your feet, focusing your attention on each part as you systematically move through your system.
- Take one minute every few hours to focus on your senses—smell, hear, feel, etc., without naming—just experience.
- Let go of focusing on a "finish line" type of goal in sex. Replace it with a goal of simply experiencing pleasure.
- Include simple ways to connect to your lover, before, during, and after lovemaking.
- Match your breathing rhythms—inhale and exhale together.
- Look into each other's eyes, softly and deeply.

Singles

Most people probably think of Tantra—and Tantric activities—as something to be done as part of a couple. And while it is true that this can be a wonderful experience for a couple to share, there are many benefits to studying Tantra as a single person as well.

The Benefits of Studying While Single

By beginning your journey to learn about Tantra while you are single, you have some advantages over those new Tantrics who are in committed relationships. For one thing, this is a period in your life when you can—and should—focus on your own internal growth and spiritual nourishment. It is fine to be "selfish" and concentrate fully on your own needs right now.

Also, by evaluating your own wants, needs, and beliefs, you will have a better idea of the type of partner you need, and the type of person who will best complement you (the perfect yin to your yang). This can save you countless wasted nights on dates with people who are not a good match for you.

Perhaps most importantly, by studying Tantra from a solo standpoint before embarking on a new, serious relationship, you will be starting from a position of power, strength, and clarity. You will have achieved self-love and self-acceptance, both critical factors in maintaining a successful relationship. As the saying goes, "You can't love someone else until you love yourself." By first taking the time to reach a happy and peaceful place in your life, you will be in prime position to start a happy beginning with someone else.

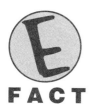

FACT

Many Tantra teachers believe it is easier to learn Tantra while single and then embark on a new relationship from a Tantric approach than it is to add Tantra to an existing relationship. This is because established relationships already have patterns and routines in place that can be tough to change, whereas with a new relationship you can start fresh.

Abandon Your "Ideal Mate" Ideas

There is another important reason why it can be helpful to explore Tantric ideas while you are single. The revelations and insight you gain through Tantra can be an eye-opener in relation to your romantic patterns and the roadblocks that prevent you from finding your soul mate. Most people go through life looking for their perfect man or woman, as they envision this elusive perfect person to be. They often limit their dating experiences to people who are their "type" and fit the preconceived image of what kind of mate they want.

This misguided strategy can be very detrimental to the process of finding happiness. Think about it: Obviously, your perfect type has not turned out to be such a great match for you, or you would not be single right now. Most likely, changing your mental image of Mr. or Ms. Right and broadening your dating horizons will prove to be a very good thing.

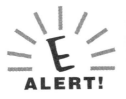
ALERT!

Keep in mind that at many Tantra events and workshops, it is common practice to pair up solo attendees with a partner of the opposite sex in order to practice various exercises and techniques. This can prove to be a valuable hands-on learning opportunity, but if it will make you uncomfortable, ask about this issue beforehand.

After exposing yourself to Tantric teachings, you may discover that you were going about this whole dating thing all wrong, taking an approach that was destined to leave you alone and unhappy. The image you have in your mind of your "perfect" mate is probably someone who in reality is totally wrong for you. Tantra may help you realize that you need to adjust your way of thinking. You will learn how to see what is truly important in a potential partner, and how to appreciate many different qualities in a person. You will also learn that many different types of people—even those who don't resemble your "perfect" mate in any way—can complement you in a way nobody else can. Who knows? You may come to the sudden realization that your true perfect partner has been right in front of your eyes the whole time, but you were not seeing clearly enough to realize it.

Couples

It can be convenient—as well as a wonderfully enriching bonding experience—for a couple to begin studying Tantra together. In addition to the positive experience of exploring something new as a couple, you will also learn an assortment of great sexual techniques and romantic rituals that you both will enjoy. In the end, most couples find this to be a rewarding journey, as well as an intimate bonding experience.

A Romance Refresher Course

The sad reality is, most people stumble through relationships blindly, at least for the first few times. You are not born knowing how to be a good lover, partner, or companion. At most, you skim through a few sex articles, whip out a candle or two, and hope for the best.

Many children and teenagers today are required to take sex education classes as part of their mandatory school curriculum. This is, of course, important from a safe sex standpoint. But these classes never cover the romantic side of intimacy—and, of course, students of that age aren't all that interested in hearing about strengthening their romantic connections.

Unfortunately, adults are not required to take any type of "Intimacy Instruction 101" course. This is really a shame, because virtually all adults could benefit from this type of education. Even those who consider themselves fairly well informed when it comes to romance are probably short-changing themselves and their partners by not taking advantage of techniques like those practiced as part of sacred sexuality rituals.

This is where Tantra (especially Neo-Tantra) can save the day. Tantra encourages people to study the sexual arts and open themselves up to learning ways in which they can improve their intimate relationships.

And since Tantra encourages couples to learn together, the partners take turns being the teacher and the student. This in itself can be a powerful bonding experience, as each partner has the chance to teach as well as to learn from the other.

Are Your Needs Compatible?

You and your partner do not necessarily have to be seeking the same exact thing from Tantra. Your specific needs or goals may differ slightly from your partner's, and that is fine. The important thing is that your needs are compatible, and that you both respect the other's motivations for this endeavor.

Perhaps you feel overburdened by stress and are worried that you have become too concerned with the material trappings of life. You pursue

Tantra mainly to benefit from the relaxing aspects of Tantric yoga, breathing routines, and meditation. Your partner, meanwhile, is more interested in the sensual side of Tantra. He wants to master the secret of sacred sexuality, so as to enhance the special relationship the two of you share.

As you both respect and support the other's motivation and are receptive to sharing in each other's newfound knowledge—and, even better, if you are open to accompanying each other to Tantra workshops and events—this can work out just fine. Although you each have separate and different goals, in the end you will both benefit from the overall experience, thanks to the stronger relationship you will have as a result of this learning process.

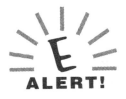

ALERT!

In contemplating what you hope to get out of Tantra, it is important to acknowledge what Tantra can and cannot do. While it can—and often does—greatly enhance a loving relationship, it is not a magic wand. If your relationship is on the rocks, it's unrealistic to hope Tantra can be a magic cure that solves your romantic woes.

On the other hand, if you plan to study the history and roots of Tantra because you have a burning desire to absorb some of Tantra's spiritual legacy and adopt the traditional beliefs, but your partner thinks all of that ancient stuff is a bunch of make-believe mumbo jumbo, this could be a problem.

Depending on how serious you are about studying Tantra, and how critical your partner is of your interest, at some point you may need to decide whether you want to pursue a relationship with someone who does not respect your attempts at spiritual growth.

When Your Libidos Are on Different Levels

Mismatched libidos—sadly, it is a common problem in many relationships, especially if the partners have been together for a while and have settled into their individual "default" settings once the frenzied "honeymoon" period has passed. Oh, how wonderful it would be if couples' libidos magically synchronized when they got together, ensuring they would always both be in the mood at the same time. Yes, that truly would be a secret to eternal bliss.

Alas, that does not happen in real life. It is rare for two people to be totally in sync when it comes to their sex drive. Even the most sexually compatible couples generally have at least moderately unequal levels of sexual desire. This is perfectly normal and nothing to be concerned about. The best way to deal with it is just to "go with the flow," accepting and even embracing your different libido levels.

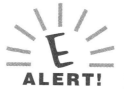

ALERT!

When discussing differing libidos, we mean that one partner's desire for sex in general is lower than the other's. This is not a reflection of their desire for their partner specifically. However, if one person does become less interested or aroused by their partner, causing the "playing field" of passion to be uneven, that is a more serious problem.

When you are starting out learning about Tantra, do not feel that your libidos must be in perfect harmony in order for this endeavor to succeed. Tantra recognizes that each person has his or her own unique needs and levels of desire. While Tantra encourages you to come up with creative ways to get your partner's engines revved up and give his or her libido a boost, it also stresses the importance of recognizing your partner's feelings and respecting the fact that he or she may not be interested in sex at a particular time.

As long as both partners can respect and understand each other's feelings and be supportive of sexual differences, things will be fine. Perhaps when the person with a lower sex drive is not in the mood for sex, he or she can encourage the other to seek alternative means of pleasure, such as masturbation or the use of sex toys. Or, as partners, you may be able to come up with some other kind of creative solution or some form of compromise. As long as it is something both parties support and are happy with, it will work just fine.

Chapter 6

Yoga, Exercise, and Meditation

Yoga, meditation, and exercise are all central topics in Tantric teachings. To truly take advantages of the benefits Tantra has to offer, you need to work these activities into your daily life. By using these tools to get your body and mind in optimal condition, you will be able to take full advantage of all that Tantra has to offer. A bonus: Being in peak mental and physical condition also spells a big improvement in your love life.

Breathing Basics

This goes without saying, but breathing is very important. It is something you must do constantly, day and night, in order to exist. It is, you might say, the most essential force of life.

Still, most people don't really give breathing much thought. They take it for granted. This is a mistake. You should consciously pay attention to how you are breathing. Tantrics believe that mastering the breath is akin to mastering the mind and spirit. Focusing on your breathing forces you to become more centered, to grow more attuned to your body and your environment.

Most people use only a small portion of their lung capacity. The biggest mistake many people make when it comes to breathing is taking quick, shallow breaths. It is much more beneficial to our physical and mental health to take deep, slow breaths.

Pranayama

In yoga, breathing is so important that there is an entire art devoted to it. This is called *pranayama*. *Prana*, or breath, is what unites body, mind, and consciousness. It is the movement of awareness. The goal of pranayama is to help the practitioner achieve calmness and focus. It is also believed to help increase vitality, promote good health, and lead to a long life.

Ayurveda and Breath

Ayurveda is a system of medicine and healing that can be traced back to ancient India. It is sometimes referred to as the "science of life" because it addresses all aspects of a healthy lifestyle and how that is impacted by nature and your environment. Ayurveda teaches that breath is the physical manifestation of our emotions; that is, your emotions directly affect your breathing patterns. In order to have better control, or *ayam*, over your breathing and thus your emotions, practice pranayama, or controlled breathing.

Tantric Yoga

Yoga plays an important role in Tantra. In fact, Tantra is sometimes called "sexual yoga." The connection dates back to the very beginning of Tantra, and many people believe that Tantra initially focused on yoga long before it ever became connected with sex.

Yoga can have many physical and psychological benefits. It helps relax the body, relieve stress, calm the nerves, and promote strength and flexibility. In addition, it helps to bring the body and mind together in harmony. Plus, it sharpens focus and awareness—both of which improve many areas of your life, including your love life.

Yoga Traditions

The word *yoga* actually means "to join together." Obviously, this is very appropriate when discussing yoga and its connection to sex. Traditionally, Tantra followers viewed sexual connections as the ultimate form of yoga. Hatha yoga and Tantra complement each other, as they not only share common historical roots, but certain physical postures and positions as well. Hatha is sometimes referred to as "the yoga of the physical body," and it is generally considered the most physically strenuous type of yoga.

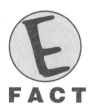

FACT

Traditionally, many Tantrics practiced hatha yoga in the nude. This was partly just for convenience's sake, simply to allow unrestricted freedom of movement. But it was also to help encourage an erotically charged atmosphere—to get the sexual energies flowing.

Kundalini Yoga

Kundalini yoga is also frequently practiced by Tantrics. This is a very spiritual type of yoga that places a heavy emphasis on meditation and breathing. Through religious practices, controlled breathing, yoga asanas (a pose or posture), and deep meditative states, the yogi can achieve altered states of consciousness. When one experiences a kundalini awakening, the life-sustaining energy that resides in the base of the spine is uncoiled and released, causing deep spiritual development.

The Benefits of Yoga

By practicing yoga regularly, you can reap many rewards in all aspects of your life. It helps relax the body, relieve stress, calm the nerves, and promote strength and flexibility. Just by lowering your stress levels, you can greatly improve your state of mind and also reduce stress-related health problems, like high blood pressure. In addition, yoga helps to bring the body and mind together in harmony. It also sharpens focus and awareness—both of which improve many areas of your life, including your love life.

But yoga can also provide some specific sexual benefits. Many yoga poses are similar to sexual positions, so by mastering the poses in a yoga setting, you become accustomed to them and are much more comfortable trying them in the bedroom. In addition, yoga promotes balance and flexibility, both of which tend to come in very handy during sex. You also gain self-awareness. This allows you to be more in touch with your emotions and more aware of physical sensations.

Solo Yoga Moves

You can do the majority of yoga postures by yourself in the comfort of your home or wherever you have some quiet, relaxing space. Following are some of the most basic one-person yoga asanas.

The Triangle

The Triangle is a stretching asana that is similar to a move that people often do while warming up for aerobics or other physical routines. Stand up straight, with feet apart. Reach up with your left arm, bend to the right. Keep your right arm on the right leg for support, allowing it to slide down your leg as you stretch further. Hold for thirty seconds or one minute. Straighten up slowly while inhaling. Repeat stretch with the other side.

The Cobra

Lie face-down on the floor with your legs straight and together. Put your hands on the floor, palms down, to support your weight. Slowly bring your head and chest up off the floor, gradually bringing them up and back, as if you were looking up at the ceiling. Stretch the upper part of your body as far back as you can comfortably, while only raising your hips off the floor as little as possible. Hold the pose for several beats and then exhale while gradually lowering your head and shoulders back to the floor.

The Butterfly

Sit on the floor and bend your legs in toward you. Bring the soles of your feet together, keeping your feet as near to your body as possible. Alternate raising and lowering your knees to the floor.

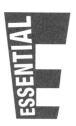

Every yoga pose actually consists of a three-step process: getting into the pose, holding it, and releasing it. The middle step is probably the most important—the longer you hold a pose, the more benefit you will generally get out of it.

The Lotus

This is the most familiar yoga pose, the one most people probably think of when they picture yoga or meditation. You sit on the floor and fold your legs in, one at a time, so that each foot is resting on the opposite thigh. This pose can be tricky for some people at first, so you may need to practice or wait until you've become a bit more limber by doing the Butterfly for a while first.

Sun Salutation

The Sun Salutation is a continuous cycle of twelve stretching moves. This is a great exercise because it involves all parts of the body, and is thus an effective all-purpose stretching routine. The steps are as follows:

1. Stand up straight with your feet together and your hands pressed together in front of you (envision a typical praying pose).
2. While inhaling, raise your arms straight above your head.
3. Exhale while slowly bringing your arms down to the floor in front of you (you can also grasp your calves with your hands).
4. Inhale and, with your hands on the floor, kick one leg out behind you, in a lunge type of movement.
5. Exhale and bring the other foot back behind you, so both legs are now outstretched behind you.
6. Inhale while lowering your hips and lower your body to the floor. You should be supporting yourself on your hands, with arms straight and head up.
7. Exhale while bending your elbows and lowering your head to the floor. You should now look as if you are about to do a pushup.
8. Continue to exhale steadily while raising yourself up on your arms. You should now be in the "raised pushup" position.
9. Inhale and bring one knee in toward your chest while keeping the other leg outstretched behind you.
10. Repeat step three, bending over and bringing your head toward your knees.
11. Inhale while lifting your arms above your head.
12. While slowly exhaling, drop your arms to your sides.

The Tree

As the name implies, you should visualize yourself as a tree—perhaps a mighty oak—with your legs and feet keeping you planted firmly on the ground. Keeping one leg straight, bring your other foot up against the straight leg, so your foot rests against the opposite thigh. Take a few deep breaths and repeat, switching legs.

The Cat

Get on your hands and knees, putting your head down while curving your back up. Envision the movement a cat makes while stretching. Hold this pose for a moment, then lift your head up while bringing your back down. Keep alternating poses slowly. This helps stretch your back and hips.

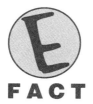

FACT

Many people find that they have great sexual encounters immediately after an intense yoga session. This is not surprising—the exercise has stimulated chemicals in the brain that boost the libido. Not to mention, the yoga session has helped you warm up and stretch out. Bottom line: You're limber, in touch with your body, and ready for action.

Couples Yoga

Yoga can be a great bonding activity for a couple to do together. It can help establish trust, encourage teamwork and cooperation, and boost your communication skills. Not to mention, it can be fun and a great stress-reducer. There are some yoga poses that are specifically designed for a couple to do together. These asanas increase one's awareness of his or her partner, increase the flow of energy between them, and heighten the spiritual awareness that goes along with love and sex.

How to Start

It is a good idea to begin a yoga session for couples with a small ritual or meditation. Here is an example:

Sit down facing one another. Put your hands together, palm to palm, and chant "Ong namo guru dev namo" three times. (You may substitute another chant if you like.) This mantra recognizes the universal creator and the teacher within. Maintaining eye contact with your partner, gently bow to each other in recognition of the wisdom and God-consciousness that he or she carries within. Radiate love and harmony. Now you may proceed with the routine.

Happy Hug

Stand facing each other with your toes touching. Now hug, releasing yourself into your partner's arms. Take five deep breaths in unison with your partner. Let the air fill your abdomen and then slowly exhale all of it, releasing your tensions, fears, and stress. Take turns rubbing each other's back for a minute or two.

Tree Together

This asana is the Tree pose adapted for couples. Stand side by side. Now, lift your outside leg up and place your foot on your inside leg's thigh above the knee. If you need to, you can support your foot with your hand. Wrap your inside arm around your partner's waist for balance and support. Make your neck as long as you can, stretching it up to the ceiling. Make your legs firm and strong, like roots buried deep in the earth. Breathe in unison and relax into the pose. After taking several deep breaths, switch sides with your partner and repeat the exercise.

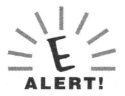
ALERT!

Warning: Many advanced yoga poses require considerable balance and flexibility. Do not be discouraged if these are difficult or impossible for you at first. Start with more basic poses and gradually work your way up to the most advanced levels.

Tantric Twist

Sit back to back, with your legs crossed. Make sure that your lower backs are touching and keep them as close together as possible throughout the exercise. Twist around to your left. Place your left hand on your partner's right knee. Place your right hand on your own left knee. Look behind you and relax your neck and face muscles, pulling firmly on your partner's knee. Take several deep breaths together. Switch directions and repeat.

Couple's Moon Triangle

This asana is a variation on the Triangle Pose. Begin by facing each other, standing with your feet as wide apart as they can comfortably be. Now place your right leg so that it overlaps your partner's left leg, so that you are no longer directly in front of each other but are facing each other somewhat diagonally. Stretch your arms out to either side of your body. Make them as long as you can. Lean over to your right side as your partner does the same. Be sure to keep your hips centered. Tip over like a teapot. Now, slide right hand down your right leg, supporting yourself just above or below the knee, never on the kneecap itself. Extend your other arm straight up toward the ceiling with palm facing inward. You should now be face to face with your partner. Look into each other's eyes. Press your palms together. Hold the position for a while, allowing your energies to flow through each other.

Couple's Lotus Pose

Since this exercise is more spiritual than physical, it is often a good way to wrap up a session. Sit in lotus pose, facing each other, with your knees touching those of your partner. Join hands and lay them in the crease between your knees, uniting you in a continuous flow of energy. Close your eyes, and concentrate on the energy between you. Imagine your energies intertwining and mingling. If other thoughts enter your mind, gently let them go. Focus only on your partner's energy. Lose yourself in your partner. This can be an impressive spiritual experience. There is no time limit. Allow yourselves to come out of it when the time feels right.

Why Exercise Is Important

Physical fitness is important for a long list of reasons—primarily because it keeps you healthy and increases the odds of a long life. From a Tantric standpoint, fitness is important because it encourages physical and mental well-being, sharpens focus, reduces stress, and improves your overall disposition. In addition, it encourages flexibility and strength, which will come in handy in the bedroom. Exercise is also important because it stimulates endorphins and other chemicals in the body that boost the libido. Many people find that exercise helps put them "in the mood."

Exercising together can also be a great experience for a couple. This topic is covered in greater detail in Chapter 18.

Meditation Basics

Many people imagine meditation as complete stillness of the mind. They imagine sitting cross-legged or in the lotus position and chanting "Om." However, there are many ways to meditate. In fact, nearly any activity can be turned into a meditative act. The secret is in not trying to block all thoughts from entering, but rather to welcome them and let them pass. Do not hold on to any one particular thought. You are in your meditative state to relax, not to fight incoming thoughts. The important thing is to avoid obsessing over problems or worrying about negative thoughts.

Getting Started

Start by finding a comfortable place without any distractions. In other words, no telephone, television, children, or chores. (This can be a challenge, but it will be worth the trouble.) Make yourself comfortable. Begin by taking deep breaths, all the way into your abdomen. Feel how your stomach expands as you inhale. Now exhale. Let all of the air out. Empty your lungs completely.

There are several relaxation techniques you can use as well. Try tightening and relaxing each part of your body one at a time, from your feet to your forehead. You can imagine inhaling light and exhaling all negativities.

Traditional Tantric Meditation Technique

Tantric meditation takes this basic meditation technique and expands upon it. Through practice, the Tantric can enter into a state of complete relaxation. From there, Tantra teaches that she or he will become conscious of the life force within. The Tantric will direct this energy from the base of the spine, up to the neck, and finally to the forehead. Tantrics can then, with experience, direct that life energy out from the forehead and form a body of energy before him or her. The body of energy will become denser and expand until reaching human size.

This body of light, which is the representation of the person's consciousness, will then become the target of their love and devotion. After half an hour or so in the meditative state, the body of light will gradually become smaller and eventually return to the person's forehead and travel down the spine. This meditation is meant to be renewing for the practitioner. It awakens energies that lie untapped at the base of your spine, providing you with a new outlook on your surroundings, your relationships, and yourself.

Health (Ayurveda)

Ayurveda teaches us to listen to the rhythms of nature and our bodies, to apply nature's wisdom to our own well-being and to that of those around us. One of the many ways that it varies from Western medicine is in its definition of health.

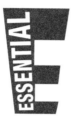

According to the Ayurveda philosophy, health is not just an absence of disease; it is achieved when there is perfect balance between all three doshas—balance between the mind, the body, and the soul.

Doshas

The Ayurveda approach believes that every person's body consists of a unique combination of fundamental energies, or *doshas*, of the mind, body, and soul. These doshas are essential to holistic health. We are all made up of unique combinations of them, which then form our individual personalities, health risks, physical characteristics, and internal workings. The particular combination of these energies creates the constitution of each person, which in today's Western terms is comparable to the genetic code. While the underlying code remains constant, external factors are in constant flux and greatly affect our balance. We may experience imbalances caused by stress, change of seasons, diet, or repressed emotions. Each type of imbalance affects each type of dosha differently.

We will not make good lovers if we are tired, stressed, and cranky. All of these moods are symptoms of a doshic imbalance. If the problem is due to an imbalance, the best way to treat it is by rebalancing the doshas. This can be done in part through the establishment of a routine. This means that you should wake up, eat, and go to bed around the same time every day. We should pay attention to our doshas and eat in a way that complements our unique makeup. It is essential that we take time out to relax, meditate, and do yoga. We can align ourselves with nature's rhythms in many different ways. However, the first step is to listen to and learn from our bodies and our surroundings. Ayurveda facilitates that process.

Unique Aspects of Ayurveda

Ayurveda differs from the contemporary, mainstream approach to medicine in several ways. For one thing, Ayurveda views each person as a unique person with unique needs. Therefore, the lifestyle, dietary guidelines, and other directives prescribed for one person may be totally different from those recommended for someone else.

Ayurveda also places major importance on the relationship between mind and body. It is believed that many health problems are caused by the mind and body not working together harmoniously as they should.

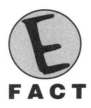

FACT

Ancient people who practiced Ayurveda believed in the strong connection between the soul and the body, especially the senses. It was believed that as the soul began preparing to leave the body, the senses would begin shutting down and the person would stop doing things (like eating favorite foods) he previously enjoyed.

Herbal products and supplements are often used in Ayurveda to help speed the healing process or to attain physical balance.

Pancha Karma

One of the most important processes involved in traditional Ayurveda was *Pancha Karma.* This was a multifaceted process designed to help establish the proper balance of mind, body, and soul. The main function of Pancha Karma was cleansing the body and getting rid of toxins. This was achieved through several techniques, many of which would be seen as unappealing or unpleasant to many modern-day people. Pancha Karma often involved vomiting to clear the stomach, enemas to clear the intestines, and a solution used to clear the nasal passages.

Chapter 7

The Importance of Environment: A Sensual Space

Your living space has a major bearing on your own personal well-being and attitude. If your environment is frenetic, noisy, and upsetting, that is bound to have a negative effect on your spirit. Likewise, a happy, soothing environment can boost the soul. This environmental connection is especially important when it comes to your sacred sensual space. If you want to set the right mood, you need to play close attention to your love nest.

Why Space Matters

You are probably already very aware of the correlation between your environment and your state of mind. Just thinking of the enjoyable aura of specific places where you feel relaxed probably has a calming effect on your demeanor.

It goes without saying that it is much easier to feel relaxed and focused when you are in a peaceful place that evokes a sense of calmness. By contrast, it can be tough to feel centered and peaceful if you are surrounded by noise, distractions, and stress. Anyone who has ever worked in a busy office—or tried to concentrate while kids were roughhousing in the same room—can attest to the importance of a calm space. Even if you had previously felt relaxed and content, entering a stressful or chaotic space will immediately increase your tensions and anxiety levels.

Space and Sensuality

All human beings need a calm space where they can retreat and recuperate from the stresses of the outside world. You need a safe haven, a place to be alone with your thoughts and escape from any negative forces. This is especially true when you are trying to create a sacred space for your lovemaking. You want a sensual space that welcomes you and your partner with a comforting feeling. This should be a place that can serve as your escape from the chaos and distractions of the world outside. It is your sanctuary where you can share your innermost secrets, private desires, and wildest fantasies with your partner without distractions or disturbances. In your sacred space, you should be able to fully concentrate on just enjoying the moments you share with that special person.

Think about how you feel when you go away to a very romantic resort or lovers' getaway. Chances are, you automatically begin to feel romantic, loving—perhaps even aroused, even if you did not feel that way before you arrived. The setting sets the spark that creates the mood. The good news is, you do not need to limit this experience to the rare times when you can head to a distant getaway. You can create your own private lovers' retreat right in your very own home.

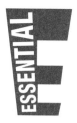

Need to create your own private pleasure palace, but don't have a lot of time? Concentrate on the big things like eliminating major distractions and mood killers. Remove the phone (or at least make sure it is unplugged), get rid of the TV, and set up some romantic, soothing candles. A few small gestures can make a big difference.

What You Will Need

Exactly what will you need in order to transform your so-so surroundings into a pleasure paradise? That can vary widely depending on your existing space, the mood you are aiming for, and your available resources. Your sacred-space shopping list can be as basic or as complicated as you wish. At the very least, you will need the bare essentials: a few soft light bulbs, some candles, something that smells good, and an assortment of "sexy" accessories.

Evaluating Your Space

When preparing to establish a sacred space, it is important to keep in mind that you do not necessarily need to designate an entire room for this purpose. (While that would be great, for many people it is simply not feasible or practical.) You can transform any room—or part of a room—into a sacred space at any time, with a little advance planning or some fast touchups. Once you have chosen the specific room or area that you will designate as your sacred space, you need to form a plan of attack and figure out how you will transform it into your Tantric temple of love. First, zero in on any major "no-nos"—things that are sure to zap the romance right out of the room. This would include a crib or your kids' toys. Yes, you enjoy being parents, but during these interludes you will want to take a break from being Mommy and Daddy. Other things that should be totally off-limits: computers, cell phones, and anything remotely connected to work.

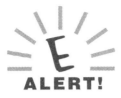

ALERT!

This should go without saying, but the very first step in preparing your sacred space is a very thorough cleaning. Get rid of all clutter. Remember, you may be trying out some adventurous positions, so you never know where you might end up sitting, laying, etc.

After you have eliminated the trouble spots, formulate your plan of action. Take your time and be creative. Is your partner turned on by burlesque shows? See if you can give your space that burlesque feeling. If your partner is more of the "wild outdoors" type, create your own little jungle paradise—complete with a few African-inspired accessories—where you can live out your "Tarzan and Jane" fantasies. For the true Tantric feel, you might want to look for a few items with an Indian influence. You will be amazed at how even a few simple touches can give the room a whole new feel—and, as a result, give you a whole new feel when you are in it.

Essentials of the Perfect Sacred Space

Everyone's sacred space should be unique. Your space will be a reflection of your own individual preferences, interests, and personality. It should be a place where you feel at home, surrounded by things that make you happy. This space should hug you and envelop you, like a well-worn comfy shoe. So there is no "one size fits all" guideline for the perfect sacred space. However, there are some critical basic aspects of the sacred space that everyone needs to consider.

The Centerpiece

The most important area of the sacred space is, not surprisingly, the bed or wherever you plan to enjoy sacred sex with your partner. This is the centerpiece, the main focal point of the entire area. It should be inviting and exciting, the focal point of the room. It also needs to be a place where you will feel completely relaxed and open to sensual experiences. Make sure the bed has comfortable blankets or spreads and lots of pillows. Some people like to drape their headboard or the top of their bed with fabric, making a tent that evokes a royal, exotic feel.

Keep in mind, though, that there is no rule that says the bed has to be the area where all the action happens. You can also arrange a love nest of blankets and large soft pillows on the floor or in a corner of the room. If you are accustomed to the normal routine of making love in your bed, just this new and exciting aspect of the sacred space can add a stimulating spark.

Lighting

One of the most important tasks when creating a sensual space is to pay attention to the lighting. Lighting makes a huge impact on our environment. Think about how hard it is to relax when you are in a room with extremely bright lights. By contrast, soft, muted lighting can make you feel calm and mellow. Lighting is especially important when it comes to a sacred romantic sanctuary. People naturally feel more relaxed when surrounded by soft lighting. (Not to mention, soft lighting is said to be more flattering and thus more comfortable for people who may be self-conscious about their body.) Buy some bulbs specifically designed to give off soft light. If you can find them in a pleasing pastel color, that is a big bonus. At the very least, dim the lights for a cozier feel. Better yet, turn off the lights completely and rely on candlelight. It's very romantic!

Use Good Scents

One of our most powerful and sensitive senses is the sense of smell. After all, it is very tough to feel romantic if there is an unpleasant smell wafting through the air. On the other hand, an enjoyable smell—or one that evokes a pleasant image or memory—can trigger excitement and arousal.

The exact smell you want will depend on your tastes and that of your partner. Many people enjoy incense, which is available in a wide range of scents. The same goes for potpourri. Scented candles are also a good choice. Flowers can also make your sacred space smell wonderful.

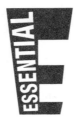

Visit your local aromatherapy store and check out the wide variety of scented oils and other aromatic treats they have to offer. You will most likely discover several new exciting scents that will be the perfect addition to your space.

Don't be afraid to do something different. If both of you are addicted to chocolate, try to find some chocolate-scented candles. (Or create your own makeshift "chocolate perfume" by placing a dish of melted chocolate near a slowly turning fan.) Perhaps the two of you have great memories of your recent X-rated romp on a tropical beach. In that case, a simple whiff of suntan lotion might be all it takes to get things rolling. Many women joke that the smell of broiling steak is a major turn-on for their man. Go with whatever works.

Don't Skimp on the Sheets

If your sacred space is in a bedroom, you should pay extra attention to the sheets. Good sheets can make a huge difference in the overall experience. Many people feel sexy when lying on silk or satin sheets. But comfort is the key here: If you (or your partner) are always cold, you actually might find a good set of flannel sheets more enticing. The main thing is to invest in at least one really good set of sheets. But don't fall into the trap of wanting to protect your good sheets. Sure, you may have spent a pretty penny on them—but look at it as an investment in your sexual happiness. Don't be afraid to "mess them up." When it comes to sheets, it's usually true that the messier they are, the more fun you've been having. So go wild—you can always wash the sheets later.

Music for Your (Sexy) Soul

Sound is another important aspect of creating a sacred space. Many people enjoy the sounds of soothing music. (There are even some CDs available specifically for Tantric rituals.) On the other hand, fast-paced music with a driving beat can get your blood pumping. Again, this will depend on your tastes. Some people enjoy jazz, while others might like the intense throbbing of heavy metal. A lot of people prefer instrumental music for romantic interludes—they find lyrics distracting and don't want to get caught singing along when they should be focused on more important things. For a peaceful, soothing mood, look for a CD that plays sounds of the ocean or forest.

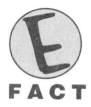

FACT

You can find many CDs designed especially for Tantric lovemaking at major Web sites like Amazon.com or Tantra.com. Or try visiting a large music store, where you can often take a "test listen" to the CD before you buy it. There are also a few musical suggestions in the Resources section of this book.

Choosing the right sexual soundtrack can really affect your romantic intensity. Some people like to adjust the music selections depending on the specific sensual activity taking place. During foreplay, many people like to go with a CD specifically designed for meditation or yoga, to encourage a leisurely relaxing pace. (Ask for these at your local record store.) While musical tastes may vary, few people enjoy getting romantic in total silence. At the very least, you might want to invest in a "white noise" machine to help block out the racket from the outside world.

Guide the Way

When preparing for a special encounter in your sacred space, it can be an exciting gesture to "pave the trail," showing your partner the way. Make a trail of rose petals, chocolates, perhaps even a few sex toys or bottles of massage oil. Better yet, arrange a series of clues that your partner needs to solve in order to figure out the route to romance. It will be like a treasure hunt—with you as the treasure, of course. For an added touch of mystery and intrigue, hang a luxurious curtain or exotic-looking scarf across the entrance to your sacred space, clearly designating the "pathway to pleasure."

Dress the Part

For the full effect, work your wardrobe into the decorating scheme of your sacred room. If you have an Asian atmosphere, donning a kimono or silk bathrobe will be the perfect touch. With a more wild space, a leather ensemble might be the perfect way to set the mood. Something loose fitting is usually more comfortable, but don't worry if the garment is slightly awkward or prickly—there's a good chance you might not be wearing it for very long. If you are feeling really ambitious, go all out and give yourself an entirely new look with some special makeup or maybe some flowers in your hair.

Change Things Up

Even the most wonderful space can become boring after a while, so be sure to make an effort to vary the surroundings occasionally. This does not need to involve a total renovation. Simply rearrange the furniture, change the lighting, or try a new color scheme. You will feel like you are in a totally different space—not to mention, you will keep your partner guessing. He won't know what to expect each time he enters the room.

A Change of Scenery

Don't have the time or money to create a totally new sacred space? No problem. Sometimes all it takes is a little change of scenery to make things seem exciting. If you want to create a magical evening, and you and your partner usually share romantic moments in the bedroom, try shaking things up by creating a temporary sacred space somewhere else—the living room, the office, or even the kitchen. As they say, variety is the spice of life, and varying your lovemaking location can certainly add some spice to your sex life.

Feng Shui and Vastu

Long before there were interior decorators to tell people how to coordinate color schemes and arrange furniture, there were ancient arts that offered guidance in these areas.

Feng Shui

Feng shui has recently become a hot new buzzword. It may seem like the latest trendy fad, but feng shui has actually been around for thousands of years, originating in ancient China. Feng shui is based on the idea of living in harmony with your environment and surroundings. If you want to observe the principles of feng shui, here are some important guidelines to keep in mind regarding your sacred space:

- The bed should be against a solid wall, and positioned in the center of two doors.
- The headboard should be aligned in a favorable direction, which is generally recommended as north.
- Some feng shui gurus believe you should not mix shapes—as in, having both square and circular furniture, for example—because it creates confusion and discord.
- Avoid having any screens or mirrors directly across from where you will be sleeping. This is believed to reflect negative energy.
- It is considered bad luck to sleep with your feet pointing toward the door.
- You should also avoid sleeping directly under a beam or rail.

Vastu

Vastu is the ancient Indian science of design and architecture. It shares some values and beliefs with Ayurveda and yoga. Many of the principles of vastu are similar to those of feng shui. For example, you should avoid circular beds and other bedroom accessories because it causes confusion.

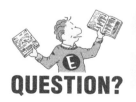

QUESTION?

What does vastu mean?
The term *vastu* comes from a Sanskrit word meaning "energy." It has also been translated to mean "a form" or "dwelling."

Vastu is often closely associated with Ayurveda, which is somewhat fitting. While Ayurveda involves the health of a person, vastu is often viewed as the art of bringing good health to buildings. Ancient people believed the "health" of a home or building had a direct profound affect on the well-being of the people inside.

Tips from an Expert

Al Link is the author of numerous books on the subject of Tantric sex, and a big believer in the importance of the perfect sensual space. Here are his tips for creating the perfect romantic environment:

Creating a sacred space is a simple, fun, playful method by which lovers can communicate to their highest and deepest levels of consciousness, in the realm of imagination and creativity, that their intention is to create a spiritual, sacred, or holy experience. This is not any ordinary quick romp in the sack. It's something special, made so by the lovers' intention. Their intention is manifested in the act of taking five or fifteen minutes to:

- Change the lighting in the room by using candles or red light bulbs that flatter skin.
- Bring in plants or fresh cut flowers.
- Drape colored cloth over sharp edges of furniture or to hide distractions such as a TV.
- Light incense or essential oils to stimulate the sense of smell.
- Arrange beautiful objects or those that have special emotional significance, like photos, mementos from trips, or romantic gifts to each other to awaken the heart.
- Present tasty tidbits of food and drink to lovingly serve each other and provide nourishment during your loving time.
- Gather a selection of music that ranges from spiritually uplifting, through romantic, to erotic, to calming, so that all your moods can be matched and enhanced.

- Array a selection of massage oils, lubricants, sex toys, so that if you want them they're easily at hand.

After the room is set up to the lovers' sensual satisfaction, ceremonies—such as the four directions ceremony—help to further purify and sanctify the space. Such actions leave no doubt that this is not just sex, but sacred sex.

Four Directions Ceremony

A four directions ceremony is a traditional ritual to bring good luck to a specific space and make it sacred. In an outdoor ceremony, smoke is often used. It is sent in all four directions while prayers and chants are spoken to sanctify the area and banish any bad spirits. Indoors, this can be done with herbs, incense, or oils—or simply be sending prayers in all four directions. Or, you can arrange four candles, setting one in each corner of the room. Walk around the room, stopping in front of each candle. Bow or kneel and say a prayer or chant asking the universe to protect the area and allow only positive energy into the space.

As you perform this ritual, you might want to keep in mind that, traditionally, each direction represents a specific element or quality:

- **East**—connected to the element of fire, which also symbolizes light and clarity
- **West**—the earth element, which can represent roots, your foundation, or strength
- **North**—air, which represents freedom and intelligence
- **South**—water, which symbolizes trust

Chapter 8

Massages, Oils, and Baths

Massage can be an incredibly romantic experience. Not to mention it is often very soothing, allowing you to leave behind the stresses of your busy day and ease into a relaxing night and perhaps some intimate encounters. This can be a very good way to reconnect romantically with your partner. Think about it: when you envision your perfect romantic evening, there's a good chance a massage appears in that scenario. But a good massage rarely just happens—you need to put some thought and effort into it. Don't worry—it will be worth it.

Massage Basics

Massage is an ancient art that has been helping people forge close personal connections for thousands of years.

People reap the benefits of massage in many ways. For one thing, all human beings need contact with other people. The power of touch can be critical to humans. In addition, massage helps alleviate stress and improves circulation. It can also help relieve sore muscles, improve skin conditions, and even improve digestion.

Massage is one of the oldest forms of preventative medical treatments. People have been using massage as a healing technique and source of comfort for thousands of years. Ancient people in China and Greece had great regard for the spiritual art of massage.

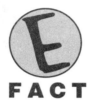

FACT

The word *massage* comes from the Greek word meaning "to knead." There are many different varieties of massage, including deep-tissue massage, sports massage, massages designed for babies, Swedish massage, and more.

In addition, massage can help alleviate physical pain and discomfort—even in areas not being massaged. This is due to the principles of acupressure and reflexology, which teach that pain in one location can often be traced back to a different part of the body, called a *trigger point* or *acupoint*. To add an extra healing and pain-relieving element to the massage, do some research on reflexology and acupressure techniques. There are many books and online resources devoted to this topic, so it should be easy to brush up on the basics.

If your partner has specific areas of discomfort or pain, you can focus a portion of your massage efforts on the corresponding trigger points. This is a very loving gesture to perform for your partner. Not to mention, your partner will be much more likely to be in the mood for love if they can get some relief from chronic pain or a nagging injury.

The Purpose of a Tantric Massage

Massage is also a wonderful way to increase intimacy and arousal. Sensual massage can be great either as an alternative to intercourse or as a prelude to sex when incorporated into your foreplay routine. The purpose of Tantric massage is not to relax (although that's a great fringe benefit) so much as it is to excite in a slow, sensual manner. It is also geared toward moving sexual energy up through the body, to awaken the higher spiritual centers. By doing Tantric massage, you awaken the body to passion and sexual awareness while at the same time strengthening the bond between you and your partner.

Put Some Planning Into It

When you decide to give your partner the gift of Tantric massage, sometimes it can add to the excitement if you make it a special event rather than a spontaneous one. Set aside a specific day and time, and make it a date. Send your partner an invitation. Perhaps you can even leave a tempting reminder on his or her voice mail, using your most sensual voice. This will keep him or her imagining the occasion, which is an essential part of the erotic process. Cancel any appointments you have at that time. Turn off the telephones and TVs and agree not to answer the door.

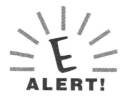

ALERT!

When getting ready to give your partner the gift of a Tantric massage, be sure to set the mood with a clean space and clean sheets. Never underestimate the importance of the proper atmosphere, especially when it comes to romance. The last thing you want to see when you make love is a pile of dirty laundry in the corner.

Have a soft blanket, pillows, and a dry towel at hand. Be sure to take some time prior to the massage to pick up some high-quality massage oil. Light candles or incense to add to the ambiance. (Tip: You may want to have a bowl of warm water and a washcloth nearby to clean up any excess oil.)

You will want to have one pillow for the head and another to place beneath the hips. Have an extra towel ready with which to cover this pillow with to protect it from oil. To prepare yourself, place a few drops of warm massage oil on your hands and move them in a circular motion to warm them up.

Sensual and Erotic Massage

You can start your massage session with a sensual massage (which differs from the sexual massage discussed later in this chapter). This can be a great way to help your partner unwind, and it can also help you gauge his or her comfort level before you attempt to proceed to a more intimate massage.

Getting Started

Have your partner lie down with his or her head on one pillow and the genitals raised by placing the pillow beneath the hips. This will enable your partner to see his or her genitals as well as your face. The legs should be spread apart and the knees slightly bent. You may even want to place a cushion beneath the knees for added support.

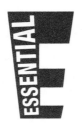

Any type of intense or prolonged massage can become tiring for the provider, and can also put a strain on hands and fingers. If your massage session lasts for a while, you should take an occasional break to stretch your fingers for a moment. Or, give your hands a short reprieve while you use your elbows or other body parts to perform the massage.

Begin by using your fingertips to gently and quickly caress the body. Use enough pressure to avoid tickling, but remember that you are not performing a deep-tissue massage here—it should be gentle. Encourage your partner to provide feedback on whether the pressure is too rough (or too soft). Be sure to maintain eye contact and take deep breaths. Ideally, this experience should be almost as relaxing for you as it is for your partner. Help your partner to continue deep breathing throughout the massage.

Focus on the Entire Body

This will be a thorough massage encompassing the entire body. Initially, you should focus on the nonsexual areas of the body, like the feet, hands, and face. This will help build the anticipation, but it will also allow you to lavish attention on parts of your partner's body that may usually get "forgotten." In the process, the two of you may discover some new territory when it comes to erogenous zones. You may realize there are some untapped "hot spots" that send little thrills throughout your body.

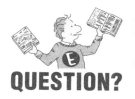

QUESTION?

Are there any special Tantric massage methods?
In keeping with the principles of Tantra, it is important to focus equal attention on both sides of the body in order to achieve balance and harmony. In other words, spend just as much time on the left side of the body as on the right. Spending uneven amounts of time on the two sides of the body may throw your partner's balance out of whack.

Be sure to take your time and show appreciation for all areas of your partner's body. While this massage often leads to sex, it should be treated as a satisfying romantic experience all of its own. You do not want to give your partner the impression that you are only going through the motions and are eager to just "get this over with" so you can move on to the main event.

Facial Massage

Many people like to wrap up their sensual massage (before moving on to the sexual massage) by massaging the neck and shoulders and, lastly, doing a facial massage. This can be very relaxing and pleasant, although men may be a bit reluctant at first, for fear of feeling like they are at the beauty parlor.

Caress all parts of the head and face, especially the temples, cheeks, and near the ears. This can help relieve stress and ward off any tension headaches. In addition, the head and face are connected to virtually every other part of the body, from a reflexology standpoint, so this part of the massage can benefit the entire body.

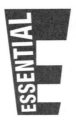

It might be helpful and interesting to study some books or Web sites dealing with reflexology. This is a science that explores the effects of massaging certain parts of the body. Reflexology establishes a connection between, for example, certain parts of the foot and backaches. By massaging specific areas of your partner's body, you may be able to alleviate his or her target stress areas.

Sexual Massage

Once you have completed your full-body sensual massage, you may want to move on to the type of massage specifically designed for sexual pleasure. These massages may be used as a prelude to intercourse, but are often done as a separate sexual activity, for the pleasure of a sexual massage is considered by many to be satisfying whether or not intercourse follows.

Lingam Massage: Just for Him

Before discussing the topic of lingam massage, it would probably be a good idea to explain exactly what is meant by the term *lingam*. Although its more broad definition refers to a stylized phallic object used in worship, in Tantric terminology it is often used as an anatomical term to refer to the penis. The purpose of lingam massage is not orgasm, although it is perfectly welcome should it happen. The purpose is to heighten sexual awareness and allow your man to let himself feel sensations that he may not have felt before. The goal is to let him relax and surrender himself to sexual and intimate pleasure. Through lingam massage, he will come into touch with his feminine side, his softer, receptive side.

Place a small amount of oil on the shaft of your partner's penis and on his testicles. Very gently massage the testicles. Be sure to be gentle; this is a very sensitive area. Massage around and above the lingam, up to the pubic bone. Now move to the perineum, found between the testicles and the anus.

Then begin to massage the shaft. Take your time here, experimenting with varying speeds and pressure. Gently take hold of the shaft with your right hand. Lightly squeezing, move your hand up the shaft and slide off. Now repeat with your left hand. Continue: right, left, right, left. Now do the same, only beginning with the head and moving down the shaft.

Place one hand at the base of the shaft. With the other, massage around and up the lingam, finishing by cupping the head. Repeat this several times. Men generally tend to like stronger, more forceful strokes than women do, so don't be afraid to be a bit aggressive. You should also keep him guessing by using a variety of movements and speeds, which will heighten the exciting sensation.

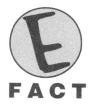

FACT

Men tend to be very visual creatures who become aroused by the sight of sex—or anything sexually exciting. To give your man an extra thrill, position him so he can watch as you give him this special massage.

To add extra excitement to your man's massage, do not limit yourself to using only your hands. Allow your hair to sweep across parts of his body, and use your breasts to stimulate one area while your hands concentrate on another.

Next stop: sacred spot. This may be an intense moment in the lingam massage. Be sure to be attentive to your partner's needs and sensations. Between the testicles and the anus, you will find a small, pea-sized spot. This is the sacred spot. Delicately press inward. He will feel the pressure deep within, which may not be very comfortable at first. With time and massage, this area will grow suppler and eventually deepen orgasms and increase control over ejaculation. Here's a tip to make the experience more enjoyable: Massage the lingam with one hand while massaging the sacred spot with the other.

Because the point of Tantric massage is not orgasm, if you feel he is about to ejaculate, ease off. Bring him to the brink and then let off. You may even try putting light pressure on the sacred spot when you feel he is near orgasm. Be aware, though, that doing this can bring strong emotions to the surface.

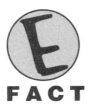

FACT

Throughout the lingam massage, he may become hard and then soft and maybe, or maybe not, hard again. This is normal and desirable in Tantric massage. You want to take him on a journey of intense highs and sensual lows. This will help him learn to be receptive and more in tune with his sexual emotions.

When you feel it is appropriate to end the massage, make sure he is comfortable and warm and let him rest for at least a few minutes.

Yoni Massage: Just for Her

The yoni massage allows your woman to relax and allow herself to enter into an excited state. So often in relationships the woman feels as though foreplay is lacking. She wishes for something more than intercourse. The yoni massage makes her feel caressed, adored, and secure, granting her the freedom and space to slip into arousal.

She will lie down as described in the lingam massage. Just as with the man, she will begin deep breathing. You will serve as her coach throughout the massage, assuring that she continues to breathe fully and deeply.

Women need to be touched and aroused before having their genitals touched. To relax her and get her ready for her yoni massage, gently caress her all over her body. Use a light touch, but not so light you tickle her. Sweep your hands over breasts, shoulders, and neck, all erotic places on a woman's body. Trace her face with your little finger and rub her scalp. When you feel she is relaxed and ready, begin the yoni massage.

Pour enough massage oil on the top of the yoni to let it drip down her outer lips and cover the outside. Begin by massaging around the yoni, on the outer lips and up to the pelvis bone. Take it slow and be sure to guide her breathing.

Take each outer lip between your fingers and gently squeeze, running your fingers up and down the outer lip. Now do the same for the inner lips.

Now we move on to the clitoris. The most sensitive part of the woman's body, the clitoris's only function is to provide pleasure. Gently stroke the clitoris in circular motions, first clockwise and then counterclockwise.

Remember that the purpose of this massage is not to reach orgasm. Simply continue the massage.

Now, using your right hand, insert your middle finger into the yoni. Gently feel around the inside. Vary the speed and pressure with which you do so. Enjoy the textures and sensations.

The next step is to locate her sacred spot. With your palm toward the ceiling, move your middle finger toward you. Using this motion, you can find the G-spot, located just under the pelvic bone and behind the clitoris. It is a spongy, tissue area about the size of a quarter. Experiment with speed, pressure, and strokes. Try circles, back and forth motions, or insert your ring finger as well. Be sure to keep looking in each other's eyes and continue deep breathing.

If you see that she is enjoying the massage, you can try placing your thumb on the clitoris and massaging the anus with the pinky. Tantra tells us that when this technique is used, "you are holding one of the mysteries of the universe in your hand."

Feel free to use your other hand to massage other parts of her body. The thumb is the best way to massage her clitoris. The sensations can be heightened by placing the rest of your hand on her mound and massaging it at the same time. Massaging the yoni with both hands, one inside and one outside, creates intense sensations, both physical as well as emotional. Keep her breathing regulated and look into her eyes.

She may, or may not, have an orgasm or even various orgasms. If this happens, be sure to maintain eye contact and continue coaching her breathing. It can be an intense experience.

When you feel that you have finished and that she is satisfied with the massage, slowly and gently remove your hands. Allow her to rest and bask in the effects of the yoni massage. Do not leave her alone. Holding her and caressing her can be tender ways to end the massage.

The Bath Ritual

The bath ritual is an important and sensual part of the Tantra massage—and, in fact, of Tantric lovemaking in general, with or without massage. Your bodies are sacred temples. During the Tantra ritual, you will be honoring and cherishing each other. A good way to show the other this adoration is by bathing. (Also, from a more practical standpoint, many people—especially women—feel more comfortable during sex if they have bathed beforehand.)

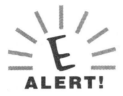

ALERT!

Be sure to spend some time preparing the bathroom before your partner arrives for the special bath. It should go without saying that the bathroom should be clean—remove all dirty clothes and linens, and give the entire room a thorough cleaning. Nothing kills the mood of a sensual bath more than dirt or mildew.

Set the mood by lighting candles and incense and playing music (but, obviously, you want to keep radios and other electric appliances a safe distance from the tub itself). For an added romantic touch, have a bottle of champagne chilling in a bucket of ice nearby. Bubbly and a bubble bath make for a great combination.

Bath salts and oils are also great additions to a sensual ambiance. Make sure the bath water is warm enough to be soothing, but not so hot as to be uncomfortable. A hot tub or whirlpool is ideal for sensual baths because of the exciting sensation of the jets hitting the skin (plus hot tubs are usually roomier and plenty big enough for two). But a regular tub can do just fine, especially if you have a massaging showerhead or bath attachment.

Wash each other with care and attention. Ideally, you should wash the entire body, including the hair (which can actually be surprisingly erotic). Use a luxurious scented shower gel or bath lotion to lather each other. Your soapy hands will be able to glide over your partner's body in new and thrilling ways. For a new and different sensation, try using a bath mitt, which you can buy at many drug stores or bath shops. Admire each other's bodies. You are preparing each other to make love, which may not necessarily mean penetration. It is part of the sensual, Tantric experience.

If you do not have a bathtub, a shower is the next best thing. What matters most is the attention you give each other.

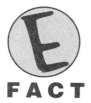

There are few Tantric sexual rituals that do not involve the required aspect of ritual bathing. This was a staple of the Tantric sex practices, and virtually all sex rituals included a bathing aspect of some kind. Most sexual rituals also involved food, wine, and massages with oils.

When you are finished bathing, apply your favorite lotions and creams. Applying the creams to your partner's body is a great way to increase the sensuality. Men, shave or trim your facial hair.

The best way to wrap up a great bath? With some warm towels, plus a cozy bathrobe or some plush blankets. Think ahead, and have these items ready for your partner when you finish your bath.

Oils

An essential part of a sensual massage is the use of oil. You can find massage oil just about everywhere—even major chain stores like Wal-Mart sell massage oil, usually near the bath supplies or personal merchandise such as condoms. Here, you can often find very affordable oils in a wide variety of types, including warming massage lotions and oils that heat up on contact.

Types of Oils

When choosing a massage oil, be sure to choose a high-quality product. Keep in mind that there are three basic types of oils: lightweight, medium-weight, and heavyweight. Light oils are moisturizing, as they are absorbed more easily into the skin. Medium oils are a bit slicker and slower to absorb into the skin. Finally, heavy oils are very slick and remain on the skin for an extended amount of time. You won't have to reapply this oil very often. It is best suited for long, Tantric massages.

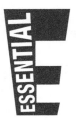

Massage oils can be great for the skin—but terrible for upholstery and linens. Keep in mind that oil can often be tough to get out of fabrics, so it is a good idea to put down an old (yet comfortable) sheet or towels to protect carpet and furniture.

Massage oils come in a nearly unlimited array of scents (and even flavors). Many people enjoy natural types of scents like vanilla, coconut, rose, lavender, or orange. But there is no one "right" scent. It is completely a matter of personal preference. Variety can be exciting, so keep experimenting with a lot of different scents and combinations of scents to find the fragrance you and your partner enjoy most. Try visiting aromatherapy shops and making your own unique scent combination.

Arousing Scents

Although it's tough to prove this scientifically, there are certain scents that are commonly believed to encourage erotic feelings and arousal. The most powerful scent connected with arousal is one you can't buy in a bottle: Human pheromones (chemicals the body releases during sexual excitement) tend to have a magnetic effect during close contact with potential partners.

Among nonbiological scents, everyone's tastes are different, so it's virtually impossible to pinpoint a single scent that will be 100 percent effective. However, scents that have been traditionally linked with arousal include cinnamon, vanilla, rose, and musky smells.

In the late '90s, Alan Hirsch, M.D., of the Smell and Taste Treatment and Research Foundation in Chicago, conducted a study to determine which scents people found most physically arousing. Of more than two dozen different scents, men showed the most aroused reaction in response to a blend of lavender and pumpkin pie. Another surprising finding: Both men and women became aroused after smelling a blend of licorice and cucumber.

Dos and Don'ts of Oils and Creams

There are some important things to keep in mind when dealing with massage oils and creams:

- Don't put oils where they are not intended to go. Keep in mind that most massage oils are not intended to go inside the body. Instead, you should use specifically designed lubricants (water-based products like Astroglide are best) for any activities involving penetration or areas inside the body. You should also take care to avoid getting any kind of oils or creams in your eyes.
- Do check the Internet, where you can find lots of "recipes" for making homemade massage oils. Experiment and find one that you like best, or be creative and come up with your own unique blend.

Chapter 9

Foreplay

When it comes to sex, foreplay often gets a bad rap. Men often complain about it, while women complain they don't get enough of it. Frequently, people of both genders view it as a chore, something necessary to be hurried through in order to get to the "main event." Even for people who give foreplay the attention it deserves, this part of sexual activity is still often seen as just the appetizer. From a Tantric viewpoint, though, foreplay can be a satisfying romantic activity all on its own.

What Is Foreplay?

Before going any further, it would probably be helpful for us to define foreplay. But that is actually easier said than done. Most people think of foreplay as the period of sexual activity (often lasting only a few minutes) that precedes the actual act of intercourse. Basically, to most people, foreplay consists of kissing, fondling, and perhaps oral sex.

The Tantric View

However, those who follow the Tantric philosophy take a different view of foreplay—one which can make it a bit tougher to define the term. Tantrics believe that foreplay can be anything which helps two people connect on a romantic level or encourages the feeling of intimacy.

Many Tantrics believe that the best approach to foreplay is to treat it not as a "warm-up" leading into sex, but rather a state of continuous affection and sensuality. In other words, a truly romantic and dedicated couple should be engaging in foreplay pretty much all of the time, by maintaining loving, considerate thoughts and performing actions that show they are always keeping their partner in mind.

Experts Share Thoughts on Foreplay

Al Link and Pala Copeland, longtime Tantra teachers, share the common Tantra view that foreplay—which can take place anywhere at any time—is a vital part of lovemaking, perhaps even more important than intercourse itself.

> *A core competency in Tantra is the ability to keep your attention fully in the present for more than a few seconds at a time. When your attention is focused in this way, you enter into a timeless space. You have nowhere to get to, nothing to accomplish, nothing that you have to do, and nothing that is forbidden. You are free. Ordinary sex typically has a goal—getting to orgasm. Reaching a goal requires a successful performance—something most lovers find daunting and intimidating.*
>
> *While Tantric sex has no goal, there is a purpose—union of the lovers and union with God/Goddess. Union is not something*

you can make happen. It requires that you surrender, letting go of any attempts to control the experience. When you understand this, foreplay becomes the main event. Each touch, caress, embrace, kiss, eye contact is complete in and of itself. They are not valued because they lead you on to something better, or more important (intercourse with orgasms), rather they are full, saturated, rich, and meaningful—each an end in itself. Ironically, when you let go of the goal of getting to orgasm you have many more of them. Over a period of hours of lovemaking Tantric lovers will typically have several sessions of intercourse, so that the total time spent in intercourse becomes a smaller portion of the time they spend together. Foreplay and after play become just as important in the total lovemaking experience.

The Importance of Foreplay

People often underestimate the importance of foreplay, or view it as simply a necessary step on the road to intercourse. This is especially true for people whose sex lives have fallen into a boring, predictable routine. They may not even really give foreplay much thought, and the foreplay period often becomes shorter and shorter as time goes by. For men especially, foreplay is something they endure (often almost grudgingly) in order to proceed to intercourse.

This, of course, is not a positive way of looking at foreplay. Foreplay is actually a critical part of the lovemaking experience, and one that should not be rushed or shortchanged. For one thing, foreplay can be an incredibly strong bonding experience that nourishes and strengthens the intimate connection between two people.

Types of Foreplay

As stated previously, the Tantra view of foreplay is that it can include anything that encourages the romantic connection between partners or builds the excitement and anticipation of an upcoming sexual encounter. But there are some common types of foreplay that you can include in your sexual repertoire.

Kissing

Many people underestimate the importance of kissing. Sure, many couples give each other an obligatory quick kiss (possibly even a peck on the cheek) upon greeting each other or saying goodbye, and perhaps even squeeze in a few other quick kisses throughout the day. But when it comes to "making out," a lot of people see that as something done only by horny teenagers or celebrities putting on a show for the paparazzi.

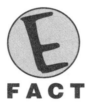

FACT

Many people are reluctant kissers, simply because they are self-conscious about their abilities in this department. Relax—everyone has the potential to be a good kisser. It just sometimes takes time to become comfortable with your kissing skills. The good news? Your partner will probably be happy to help you practice.

However, kissing—meaning the intimate, soulful, deep kind of kissing—can be a very special romantic activity. Couples who previously skimped on the kissing often discover that it is a real boon to their intimate connection. And once they enjoy a few episodes of intense kissing, most couples are hooked permanently. The key is to take your time and really enjoy the power of passionate kissing. Cherish the experience of kissing as a wonderful experience all on its own, not necessarily Step 1 of the 1-2-3 process leading to sex.

Many people mistakenly believe that kissing is a very cut-and-dry process: Pucker up and smooch your lips together. In reality, there are actually many different ways to kiss—and it can fun for you and your partner to try as many as you can think of. Try taking things very slow and exploring each other's lips and mouth. Or see how long you can engage in deep kissing without using your tongue.

Of course, kissing does not always involve two sets of lips. You can try kissing your partner on the neck or other parts of his or her face. You can also lick or nibble your partner's ears, throat, or pretty much any other part of his or her body.

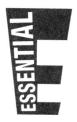

To really enjoy the experience of kissing, try sneaking in a passionate "make-out session" during a few stolen moments in the car, between meetings, or when you can grab some other short burst of time. Not only will the time limit add to the excitement, but you will also realize that kissing can be independently exciting even when it isn't followed by sex.

Oral Sex

Probably the most obvious form of foreplay is oral sex. Even in today's more sexually liberated times, many people still have a problem with oral sex. For some, the problem traces back to early misinformation about sex, or warnings from parents or other adults that oral sex is "bad" or "wrong." Other people avoid oral sex because they fear it may be gross or distasteful, or maybe even because they are afraid they won't do it correctly.

The good news is, oral sex is fun and "good." It is also something that most couples do, so it definitely isn't weird or freaky. It's also an acquired taste, in that you can learn to like it more and more.

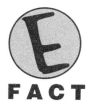

FACT

There are many ways to make oral sex more appealing to the senses. If you're worried about embarrassing tastes or smells, it can be helpful to engage in a bath ritual beforehand. Flavored and/or scented gels and lotions (be sure to make sure they're edible) can also be a big help.

Fellatio

Here's a not-very-surprising fact: Almost every man in the world loves fellatio. By treating your man to this sexual treat (known as "playing the flute" in Tantra lingo), you can give him a great gift he will really appreciate. If you are nervous about your skills, try watching a few adult films and pay attention to the fellatio techniques involved.

There is no one "right" way to perform fellatio (although one cardinal rule is to be very careful with your teeth—no biting!). Each man has his own unique likes and dislikes when it comes to the perfect fellatio technique. A lot of men enjoy the "deep throat" approach where you take his penis as far into your throat as you can comfortably handle.

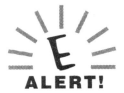

ALERT!

In a survey conducted by *Cosmopolitan* magazine, almost one-third of men said the biggest mistake women make when performing fellatio is not using her hands. In addition, 18 percent said the woman didn't suck hard enough and 11 percent were disappointed that the woman didn't pay enough attention to the testicles.

The head of the penis is particularly sensitive, so spend time licking this area and teasing it with your tongue. For enhanced pleasure, caress his testicles while performing oral sex—or you can lick them or (gently) suck on them, which will drive your man wild.

Tip: Being visual creatures, men get extremely aroused by watching you pleasure them. Position your man so that he gets a good view of you while you perform fellatio. It can be really sexy to maintain eye connect with your man while you go down on him, making it clear that you are thoroughly enjoying the act.

Cunnilingus

Cunnilingus (or "polishing the pearl" in Tantric lingo) can really drive a woman through the roof. However, many women are hesitant to try it for the first time, either because they were taught as girls to believe it is "bad" or because they are self-conscious about how their body tastes or smells. Reassure your woman that this is a natural act, perfectly allowed among consenting adults. You should also make sure she knows that you love her body and are turned on by the way it tastes and smells.

Even if she is reluctant at first, your woman will be extremely glad she tried cunnilingus once she does. The majority of women experience orgasms through oral sex, often much more easily than through intercourse.

Just as with fellatio, there is no one right way to perform cunnilingus. However, for most women, it is best if you ease your way into it, starting with her thighs or outer labia and making sure she is aroused (and lubricated) before working your way to the clitoris.

Proceed slowly once you get to the clitoris. Be alert for cues from your partner as to what feels good and what doesn't. Some women like intense, prolonged clitoral stimulation, while other women find this painful to that sensitive area. For many women, the area slightly to either side of the top of the clitoris is the most sensitive, so you might want to pay special attention to these spots.

Fondling

Fondling is another common foreplay technique. This can vary from caressing your partner's breasts to stimulating each other's genitals by hand. Since "copping a feel" is often something done when you are afraid of getting caught (imagine two teenagers behind the bleachers), this can have an added element of naughtiness to it.

Massages and Baths

In Chapter 8 you learned all about the importance of massages and baths. While they can be exciting experiences all on their own, massages and bath rituals can also both be great forms of foreplay. They also have the added benefit of relieving stress and helping you achieve a relaxed state more conducive to a great sexual experience.

Manual Stimulation

Another common foreplay activity involves manual stimulation (to put it bluntly, a hand job). This can often be synonymous with the sexual massage described in Chapter 8. However, a "hand job" is generally more aggressive and intense—think fast and furious—than the more leisurely sexual massage. Since many men can easily achieve orgasm through manual stimulation alone, this can also be a satisfying alternative on occasions when the couple can't (or simply doesn't want to) have actual intercourse.

Some women are self-conscious about their manual stimulation technique, but it is actually a pretty easy skill to master. The key is paying close attention to your partner's feedback and tailoring your technique according to the reactions (both verbal and nonverbal) you get from your partner. Most likely, it will be pretty easy to determine if your partner likes what you are doing.

The most common basic approach to stimulating a man with your hand is using rapid up and down strokes while grasping the penis with one hand. You would generally start out slowly and increase the speed and strength of your stroke as your partner becomes more aroused. However, to keep things from getting boring, you should mix things up often. Try using both hands, or alternating fast and slow strokes. You can also try a twisting move, rotating your hands back and forth around the penis.

Of course, it is also common for a man to stimulate his female partner by hand. This would generally be very similar to the yoni massage as described in Chapter 8. Many women find it arousing for their clitoris and/or vagina to be stimulated manually while kissing their partner, or while their breasts are being stimulated orally by their partner.

Simultaneous Masturbation

Masturbation is traditionally thought of as something done as a solo act, often in secret while nobody else is around. But it can be exciting (not to mention educational) to masturbate in front of, or in tandem with, your partner. This is especially exciting for men, who often find it very arousing to watch a woman pleasure herself—as evidenced by the countless adult movie scenes showing a woman masturbating.

Simultaneous masturbation can be extremely enlightening, and it can give you valuable insight into how your partner likes to be touched. Take turns watching each other masturbate (admittedly, you may feel a bit embarrassed or uncomfortable at first, but most likely it'll become such a turn-on that your inhibitions become a distant memory). Pay attention to how and where your partner touches herself. This can give you a veritable roadmap as to how to lead her into ecstasy. Take mental notes and follow that lead when it is your turn to pleasure your partner.

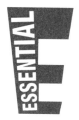

Simultaneous masturbation can help people who are reluctant to give blunt instructions in the bedroom for fear of appearing critical or bossy. By allowing your partner to watch you in action, you indirectly tell him how to please you without the risk of hurting his feelings or making him self-conscious about his existing techniques.

Fun and Games

You can also try making your foreplay more exciting by including some fun and games. In Chapter 16 you will learn more about props, toys, and other items that can be incorporated into your foreplay routine.

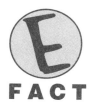

A study conducted by Durex found that people worldwide spend 19.7 minutes on foreplay, with men claiming to spend more time than women—20.2 and 18.8 respectively. The study found that the British spend the most time on foreplay, followed by Germans and the Irish, while the Thais spend the least amount of time on foreplay.

Unleash Your Inner Exotic Dancer

Try spicing up your foreplay encounter by putting on a sexy striptease for your partner. Put on some sexy music and slowly undress while doing your sexiest dance moves. This can be a great way to build anticipation and "tease" your partner. Take your time, and remind your partner that they can look, but not touch. This may seem more natural for women—but men shouldn't be afraid to do a little dance for your woman, either.

If you want to perfect your routine before putting on a performance for your partner, pick up one of the striptease instruction videos available at most adult stores or at lots of sites online. In many cities, you can find "strip-aerobics" classes, where you get the added bonus of burning lots of calories while polishing your moves.

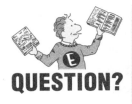

I'd like to do a striptease but I feel so self-conscious, any suggestions?

You think your partner would love watching you strip, but you feel a little embarrassed? Don't worry: This isn't a dance competition. Your partner won't be critiquing your steps. This is a situation where enthusiasm is really all you need. Your partner will be so grateful for your effort—and turned on by just about any dance moves you have—that things are bound to heat up.

Other Types of Foreplay

There are many other activities you can add to your foreplay menu. Try having an indulgent meal—perhaps including some of your favorite aphrodisiacs at a romantic restaurant. (And yes, playing footsies under the table is allowed.) Many people also find dancing to be an exciting part of foreplay. Go see a sexy movie together, and hold hands or make out like teenagers. Better yet, steam up the car windows at a drive-in.

Foreplay Talk

Talking can be a real turn-on and a great part of foreplay. But we're not referring to talking about paying the electric bill or discussing little Timmy's orthodontist appointment. That kind of talking is far from sexy and can really put a damper on a romantic evening. The talking that enhances foreplay is the "whispered sweet nothings" kind. Take time for some pillow talk, where you tell your partner how sexy she is, how much you worship him, how aroused she makes you, etc.

It can also be very exciting to give your partner a preview of the exciting things to come. Tell your partner—in explicit tantalizing detail—exactly what you intend to do to her or him as the night progresses. This will build the anticipation and help get your partner aroused.

Another type of exciting foreplay talk? Fantasy sharing. Revealing your secret sexual fantasies can be very exciting. Take turns describing your most exciting fantasies.

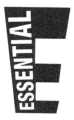

Exchanging secret sexual fantasies can be a thrill, but establish a sense of trust first. Set some ground rules, such as that neither of you will ever criticize or make fun of the other's fantasy, no matter how shocking it may be. And always hold this information confidential. Never betray your partner's trust by disclosing their fantasies to anyone else.

Many people are hesitant to disclose their fantasies, for fear that their partner will laugh—or, worse, be shocked or disgusted. So you may need to coax your partner to open up about this.

Remember that there is a big difference between fantasy and reality—just because you find the thought or image of a particular activity arousing does not mean you actually want to carry out that scenario. For example, some people find it arousing to imagine having sex with a person of the same sex—but this does not necessarily mean they really want to engage in same-sex activities in real life. The same goes for fantasies involving group sex. (Some women may be reluctant to disclose these types of fantasies for fear their partner will then pressure them to carry out the actual activities, so it is important for you to reassure your partner that you can treat her fantasies as exactly that: fantasies that will not necessarily translate into real life action.) There is some middle ground here, though. For example, if your partner fantasizes about group sex but does not actually want to engage in it, you might suggest that he or she would be turned on by watching an X-rated film involving group sex.

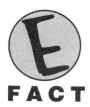

An ABC News survey found young people are more likely to discuss fantasies with partners (71 percent of those ages 18 to 29 did, compared with only 49 percent of those 40 to 49). In addition, 21 percent of respondents fantasized about a threesome, while 10 percent fantasized about having sex at work. Surprisingly, 30 percent fantasized about cheating on their partner, although only half of those admitted to actually being unfaithful.

Twenty-Four-Hour-a-Day Foreplay Ideas

As mentioned earlier in this chapter, Tantrics believe that foreplay is a continuous thing that can occur at any time, not just right before intercourse. In Tantra, couples engage in foreplay virtually nonstop, by always making their partner feel special and doing little intimate gestures for each other. Here are some ways you can engage in foreplay at any time:

- Send love notes. Leave a little sexy note (you decide how racy you want to get) in your partner's pocket, briefcase, or purse. Include a little teaser about what you plan to do to your partner during your next in-person encounter. If you're feeling really risqué, perhaps you can tear a photo from an adult magazine blatantly illustrating exactly what you want to do with your partner—perhaps with a Post-It note saying, "Can't wait to try this with you!"
- Leave your partner a little "gift basket" of her or his favorite indulgent foods (especially aphrodisiacs) and perhaps a few naughty surprised like massage creams or adult toys.
- Call your partner at random times during the day, just to say hi and let them know you are thinking of her or him.

Singles and Safe Sex: Fun with Foreplay

Sexually speaking, this is a great time to be single. People of both genders are more comfortable with their sexuality and enjoy more freedom to engage in sexual relationships—with or without the confines of a long-term relationship. However, this is also a time when safe sex is absolutely crucial. Sadly, singles today can't afford to engage in the wild, reckless abandon that was common in the "free love" 1960s and 1970s.

This is why foreplay is so perfect for sexually cautious singles. Foreplay can be satisfying while at the same time carrying relatively little risk. Most foreplay activities—such as fondling and mutual masturbation—involve no exchange of bodily fluids, making this a safe type of sexual activity. (Plus, there's the added advantage of no pregnancy worries.)

Obviously, it is still wise to practice safe sex and be prepared with condoms, finger cots, and/or latex gloves for any activities where you feel safety measures are necessary.

Foreplay Dos and Don'ts

Foreplay is a time to be adventurous and creative, so there are very few hard-and-fast rules. But there are a few general guidelines that might be helpful to keep in mind:

- Don't underestimate the importance of foreplay. This is a critical part of your relationship and a great way to strengthen your intimate connection. Never view it as a chore.
- Do maintain a lot of variety in your foreplay routine. It should never get so predictable that it falls into the Step 1, Step 2, Step 3 type of pattern.
- Don't look at foreplay as an "opening act" for intercourse. Often, foreplay can be a satisfying experience all on its own.
- Don't keep score when it comes to foreplay. It's not a case where if one partner gets ten minutes of his or her favorite foreplay, the other needs an exact amount. Foreplay should flow naturally and be flexible according to each partner's needs and wants.

Chapter 10

Kama Sutra and Sexual Positions

When discussing sexual positions, it probably makes sense to start with the basics of the Kama Sutra, the most well-known of all the sex guides. The positions in the Kama Sutra might be considered "oldies but goodies." In addition to the positions described in the Kama Sutra, there are many other positions that can be fun and exciting, but are still basic enough for most people to master relatively easily. The positions in this chapter should give you a good start in your Tantric sex journey.

The Kama Sutra

The Kama Sutra is an ancient Hindu text believed to have been written by a scholar named Mallanaga Vatsyayana. It was designed to be a manual of techniques for improving one's relationships and sexuality, and also to improve the person's overall character.

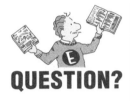

QUESTION?

Why doesn't the Kama Sutra contain more Tantric information and techniques?
Some people speculate that Vatsyayana was deliberately selective about which material he did—and did not—include in this book. Those in this camp believe he only revealed what he thought should be shared with the general public, but withheld the real Tantric mysteries, in keeping with the tradition that those closely guarded secrets should only be passed down orally from guru to student.

The Kama Sutra is based on two sets of "Sixty-Four Arts." One set of arts dealt with sex and lovemaking. This is what most people tend to think of when you mention the Kama Sutra.

But many people do not realize that the Kama Sutra also discussed the other set of Sixty-Four Arts: skills and interests felt necessary for a person to become a well-rounded, cultured person. These would include singing, theater, science, literature, and so on. The Kama Sutra even dispenses fashion advice, dictating that a woman should dress in impressive and colorful ensembles when approaching her husband—and adding that a woman should reserve her best clothes for trysts with her husband, and vice versa.

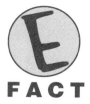

FACT

The term *Kama Sutra* roughly translated means "sensual book." In addition to dealing with sex and sexual positions, it also gives tips on dating, kissing, aphrodisiacs, and achieving orgasms. It also covers the more painful (or erotic, depending on your viewpoint) techniques of scratching and biting during sex—going so far as to categorize numerous different types of bites and scratches.

Space limitations make it impossible to cover every Kama Sutra position here. (For a more detailed look at the Kama Sutra, check out some of the books specifically dealing with that topic that are listed in the Resources section of this book.) This chapter does, however, cover some of the most popular Kama Sutra positions. You should be able to master most of them fairly easily (besides, practicing is half the fun).

Man on Top

The man-on-top position is one of the oldest sexual positions and probably the most common. For many couples, it is their "default" position, the one they automatically rely on when one or both partners are feeling particularly energetic or adventurous.

Basic Man-on-Top: Missionary Style

The basic man-on-top position—commonly known as "the missionary position"—involves the woman lying on her back, typically with her knees bent and pulled up slightly. The man gets on top of her, supporting most of his weight with his arms (the rest of his weight is supported by the woman's body). Often, the woman will wrap her legs around the man's body, sometimes interlocking her feet behind his back, especially as she becomes more excited.

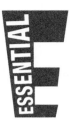

Famous sexual researcher Alfred Kinsey found that the wide majority (more than 90 percent) of married women said they used the missionary position most often. Interestingly, almost 10 percent of married women said they *only* used this position.

In conservative cultures, it is common for the man to rarely—if ever—see the woman totally naked. The missionary position is a popular choice in these situations, as it allows couples to have sex simply by lifting up the dress or skirt, or possibly even by the man inserting his penis through a gap or opening in the woman's clothing. This position is also favored in societies where it is seen as important to emphasize the man's superiority over the woman.

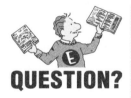

How did the "missionary position" get its nickname?
Nobody really knows for sure. There was a legend (now generally considered untrue) that, in an effort to discourage sexually adventurous behavior, early missionaries declared this the only "approved" position accepted by the church for procreation. The term first appeared in English dictionaries in the late 1960s.

Women tend to either love the missionary position or hate it. Some women like being "covered up" or shielded by the man's body, so they do not feel as vulnerable or exposed as they might in other positions. This may especially be true if the woman is self-conscious about her body. Some women also like the fact that, in this position, the man does virtually all of the work. Lastly—but perhaps most importantly—this position is one of the best for intimacy, pillow talk, etc, because of the face-to-face contact.

On the other hand, there are women who find this position uncomfortable and stifling. They may feel like they are trapped under the man. This position can also be uncomfortable for the woman if the man is especially large or heavy. One of the main drawbacks of this position, though, is that many women find it tough to reach orgasm solely through sex in this position.

Yawning Position

In one popular variation of the man-on-top position, the woman lifts her legs wider apart, bringing them up and over the man's arms. This allows for deeper penetration. This position is known as the "yawning position."

Legs Raised High (Rising Position)

A more challenging version of the yawning position involves the woman extending her legs straight up so that her feet rest on the man's shoulders (or chest). This allows her to use the man's body as leverage so she can thrust and move her hips more easily. Many women enjoy the deep penetration this position allows, although it can strain the legs if continued for a long period of time, especially if the woman is unaccustomed to being in this position.

For another variation of the legs high position, the woman puts both of her legs on the same side of her partner—meaning, both feet would be resting near a single shoulder. This position can allow for deeper penetration.

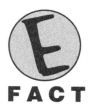

FACT

The yawning, legs raised high, and splitting the bamboo positions are all said to be very conducive to G-spot stimulation. The woman can encourage this by rotating her hips and guiding the man into the best position for maximum G-spot contact.

Splitting the Bamboo

A more challenging variation of the legs raised high position is called *splitting the bamboo*. In this position, the woman only keeps one leg fully extended to the man's shoulder. The other leg is kept bent at her side or lying flat on the bed or floor. The woman then alternates, switching legs at certain intervals (switching legs rapidly can be challenging, but the friction provides an exciting sensation).

Woman on Top

Another popular type of sexual position involves the woman positioned on top of the man. Many women—especially modern women comfortable with their sexuality—prefer the woman-on-top positions best. For one thing, some women find this position to be a real power trip. They like the idea of being in a dominating position over their man.

From a physical standpoint, this position is much more conducive to female orgasms than the missionary position. There is greater freedom of movement, allowing the woman to guide the man into a position that feels best for her.

In addition, the woman and/or her partner can stimulate her clitoris manually while in this position. Since the woman does most of the moving and thrusting in this position, she can set the pace and keep things moving at the rate she likes most. She can also take greater control over the angle, rhythm, and speed of movement, so she can find the perfect combination for maximum clitoral and G-spot stimulation.

For men, probably the greatest appeal of this position is the great view they get of their partner's breasts. Plus, a lot of men enjoy this position because it gives them a break, since the woman does most of the work. In addition, it can be exciting for a man to see his female partner in the "dominant" position. It also helps men delay ejaculation because they can relax more in this pose instead of actively thrusting.

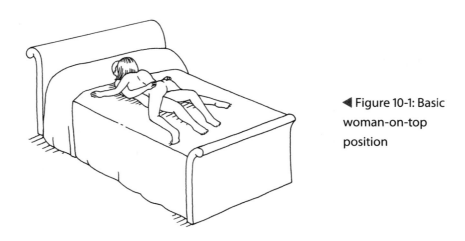

◀ Figure 10-1: Basic woman-on-top position

The basic woman-on-top position involves a man lying flat, with his legs either straight or with knees slightly bent, and the woman on top of him, so they are facing each other. The woman generally keeps her upper body raised, so she is almost in a sitting position, similar to if she were riding a horse. This position is sometimes referred to as the *inverted missionary* or the *cowgirl* position.

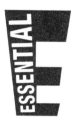

For maximum pleasure, the woman should use her hands and knees to support her weight as she lifts herself up and down off of the man's body. She should raise and lower herself at varying speeds and to varying heights for a wide range of pleasurable sensations for herself and her partner. In the Kama Sutra, this is known as the "Fluttering and Soaring Butterfly."

Other Woman-on-Top Positions

There are only three woman-on-top positions mentioned in the Kama Sutra. These are "Pair of Tongs" (the position mentioned above), the "Top" or "Bee" (where the woman turns around completely, so she is facing her lover's feet), and the "Swing" (where the man lies on his back, raises his hips in a pelvic lift and the woman sits astride him; in a more vigorous variation the man would do a complete back bend). The Kama Sutra also mentions the "Mare's Trick," which is the skill of squeezing vaginal muscles during intercourse. Woman-on-top was considered unnatural by followers of the Kama Sutra and many people who lived during the period when it was written, a naughty rarity if lovers were curious or if a man was tired out and the woman not yet satisfied. Woman-on-top was referred to as "woman acting the part of the man."

Rear Facing

Many people enjoy the rear-facing (also known as *rear entry*) positions. This is where the man is in back of the woman and enters her from behind. These positions offer several advantages. First, they make it easy for the man to use his hands to explore the woman's breasts, buttocks, and other parts of her body—including the all-important clitoris. Or, the woman can use her own hands to stimulate these parts of her body herself. At the same time, the woman can easily reach down and caress the man's penis and/or scrotum while he is entering her in this position.

Men also like this position because they have easy access to their partner's buttocks, should they wish to give her a light smack on the butt—or a harder spanking, if both parties are into that sort of thing.

Along these same lines, it also provides a good way to segue into anal penetration (either with the finger or penis)—again, assuming both parties are agreeable.

Doggie Style

Often, rear-entry positions of all variations are lumped into one general category and referred to as the "doggie style" position. But there are actually lots of slightly different variations of rear-entry positions. The Kama Sutra depicts the "dog" position as the woman on all fours, with the man behind her, grabbing her around the waist.

Elephant Style

The elephant position somewhat resembles the dog position, except the woman lies fully stretched out flat on her stomach with the man stretched out along her back. Many women automatically go from the doggie style pose into this position at a certain point as the action intensifies. An advantage is that it is easier for the woman to reach back to the man's body, which allows her to touch his legs or scrotum. This position allows for maximum penetration and stimulation of the clitoris, and many women find they are able to climax this way.

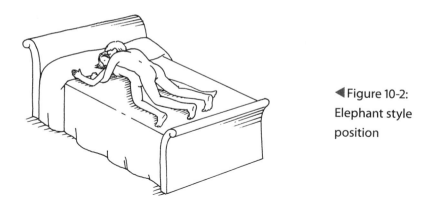

◀Figure 10-2:
Elephant style
position

Standing

Another category of lovemaking is the standing positions. One major advantage of these positions is that both parties are supporting their own weight (for the most part, anyway), which can be a big help for couples where one partner is larger/heavier than the other—or in cases where one partner has a medical condition or injury that prevents him from being able to support his partner's weight.

Standing Face-to-Face

Many couples are not very fond of having sex while standing face-to-face. For one thing, this can be difficult or virtually impossible for couples with a big height difference. Since the woman is standing up straight (as opposed to bending over, as she would with the rear-entry version), penetration can be a challenge, especially if the man is taller than her. It sometimes helps if the woman lifts one of her legs up, or if the man can lift her up slightly.

Standing Rear Entry

The standing rear-entry is a position many couples enjoy, although it can be a bit tricky, especially if there is a considerable height difference.

This may require the couple to employ a little creativity, perhaps by having the woman stand on top of a sturdy object—or, if the woman is light enough, the man may even be able to lift her up and hold her in the proper spot.

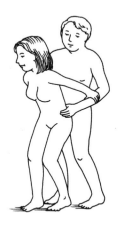

◀ Figure 10-3:
Standing rear-entry
position

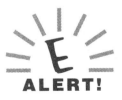

ALERT!

Try doing the standing rear-entry position while in front of a mirror. Many people (especially men) enjoy the visual stimulation of watching themselves caress their partner's breasts or other parts or her body—or watching her do this herself—while having intercourse in this way.

The Benefits of Basic Positions

Upon hearing the title of this category, some people may mistakenly assume "basic" automatically equals "boring." Nothing could be further from the truth. (And, in fact, diehard Tantrics will often say that no position is boring, as long as the partners are enthusiastic enough.)

Basic is simply a term used to mean the positions are relatively uncomplicated and easy enough for the vast majority of people to handle easily. Many people like basic positions because they do not require a lot of excess preparation or the considerable strength and/or stamina needed to tackle more advanced maneuvers.

There can be many reasons to incorporate some additional basic positions into your bedroom repertoire. Perhaps you are simply seeking a few new moves in addition to (or as an alternative to) the offerings of the Kama Sutra. Yet you may not yet have enough confidence or bravery (not to mention physical dexterity) to attempt some of the advanced positions. So these basic moves can spice up your love life but aren't too intimidating for the less adventurous crowd.

Woman on Top Variations

As mentioned in the previous chapter, the Kama Sutra actually only addresses a few woman-on-top positions. But since the woman-on-top category of positions is becoming increasingly popular today, there are many other variations on this basic theme that couples can have fun trying. Unfortunately, modern lovers cannot necessarily take credit for these enjoyable moves. It is believed some of the following positions may have been inspired by those found in ancient Indian, Arabian, or Asian texts.

Asian Cowgirl

The Asian cowgirl position involves the woman squatting on top of the man, rather than being on her knees. This can be tricky because the woman doesn't have as much support, and all of her weight is resting on the man. It can also quickly prove uncomfortable for both partners.

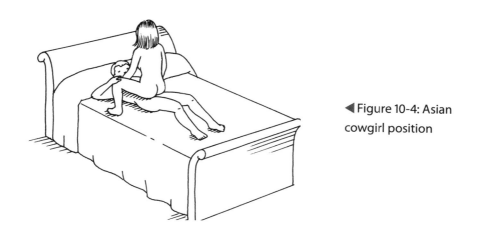

◀ Figure 10-4: Asian cowgirl position

Leaning Forward

For a more intimate feeling while in the woman-on-top position, the woman can lean forward and bring her face close to the man's. This allows for kissing and talking, and also varies the sensations of intercourse. Obviously, she should only lean forward as far as it remains comfortable to the man. Occasionally, the man will find it uncomfortable or even painful if the woman leans too far forward during sexual intercourse while on top of him.

Leaning Back

In this position, the woman leans back toward the man's knees. The woman supports herself with her hands and arms, which can make this position tiring for the woman after a while. But this position allows for greater freedom of movement and exploration possibilities—and also provides the man with an enjoyable view—so many couples find it exciting. She should lean back slowly, until she confirms how far back she can go without making the man physically uncomfortable.

Reverse Woman-on-Top

A variation of the basic woman-on-top position involves the woman sitting on top of the man with her back to him, so she is facing his feet. In the basic version of this position, the woman is supporting her weight on her knees, similar to if she were kneeling.

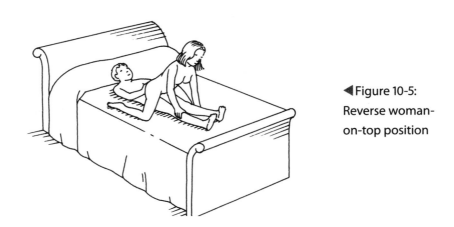

◀ Figure 10-5:
Reverse woman-
on-top position

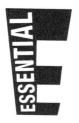

The reverse woman-on-top position is also known by a variety of other nicknames. You may hear it referred to as the "reverse cowgirl," the "reciprocal view of the posterior," or even "the reverse Amazon."

If you are really dexterous, you can try starting out in the basic girl-on-top position and then—while your man is still inside of you—spinning around to the reverse cowgirl position.

The Swan Sport

A variation of the reverse woman-on-top involves the woman on top of the man, facing his feet, with her knees bent and drawn up so her feet are flat on the bed at the man's sides. She would then thrust her hips rapidly.

Sitting Positions

In lovemaking, sitting positions offer the advantage of being very intimate, because the partners are locked together in close contact, often in an embrace type of hold. These positions are also less physically strenuous, so they are easier to maintain for long periods of time. These positions are often favored in situations where the man wants to remain aroused for a long period of time while delaying orgasm, as the couple can stay still for a while yet still remain joined in intercourse.

Yab Yum

The most common sitting position is the yab yum. This is also probably the most common and most well known sexual position associated with Tantra. This position is seen as the most conducive to allowing the partners to align their chakras. Note: This exact position is not in the Kama Sutra, but is similar to the "Embrace of Milk and Water."

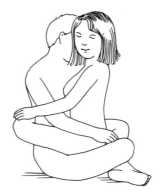

◀ Figure 10-6: Yab
yum position

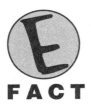

FACT

Yab yum is a basic Tantric sexual position, but it is also a term that is sometimes used to refer to lovemaking or the sexual union. The idea of yab yum is also comparable to the Chinese concept of yin and yang.

To get into this position, first the man sits down cross-legged. Then the woman sits on top of him, facing him and wrapping her legs around his back. Because the couple can embrace closely and the face-to-face contact encourages kissing or shared whispers, many people find this to be a very intimate position. However, it really isn't conducive to a lot of freedom of movement or major thrusting.

Modified Yab Yum

Some people find the yab yum position physically uncomfortable. This is especially true for people with back problems. They may prefer to do a modified version of the yab yum, in which the man sits on the edge of the bed or on a chair with his feet on the floor. The woman then sits on the man's lap, facing him.

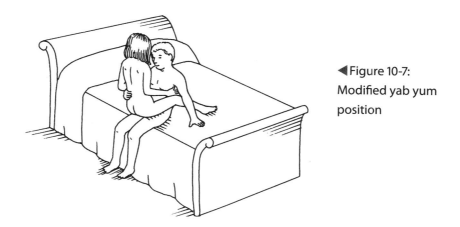

◀Figure 10-7:
Modified yab yum
position

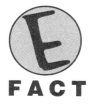

FACT

One advantage of sitting positions is that they can be performed in confined spaces. As a result, some couples like to engage in sitting positions while in new or different environments, such as in a parked car. From a distance, any onlookers may think the couple is simply embracing, assuming they have remained at least partially clothed.

Sitting Facing Same Direction

Another sitting position involves both partners facing the same direction. The man would sit down—usually on the edge of a bed, couch, or chair—and the woman would sit in his lap, with her back to him. The woman would then move herself up and down while on top of the man.

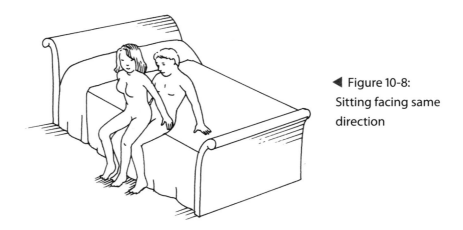

◀ Figure 10-8:
Sitting facing same
direction

Rear-Facing Variations

In addition to the rear-facing positions mentioned previously, there are other positions of that type. They are not part of the Kama Sutra, but can still be fun to try.

Both Kneeling

One of the easiest rear-entry positions involves both people sitting on their knees and leaning back—with their legs folded underneath them—on the bed or floor, with the man pressed up close behind her.

Frog Jump

Here's a creative variation of the rear-entry technique. The man kneels on the bed or floor and the woman squats down in such a way as it seems like she is about to do a frog jump. She then lowers herself onto the man and he enters her from behind. This is somewhat tricky, so it is not a position that most people can sustain for very long.

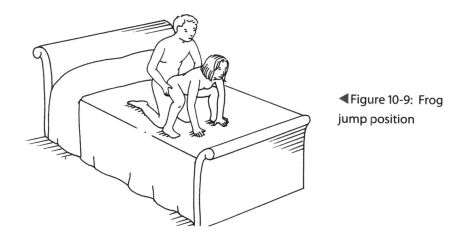

◀Figure 10-9: Frog
jump position

Other Positions

Still craving more variety but not quite ready to tackle the advanced positions yet? No problem. Your choices are limited only by your imagination. There are some other positions that you might want to try:

Scissors

The couple lies on their sides, with the man behind the woman and at a slight angle away from her. They then intercross their legs (she puts one of her legs in between his) so that they resemble a pair of scissors. This position allows for clitoral stimulation by the woman or her partner.

The Screw

The man kneels on the floor beside the bed (or stands, depending on the height of the bed). The woman lies on her side on the bed, with her knees drawn up toward her chest. The man enters her while she lies on her side. The creative penetration angle provides some unique sensations, and this position also is not very strenuous, especially for the woman.

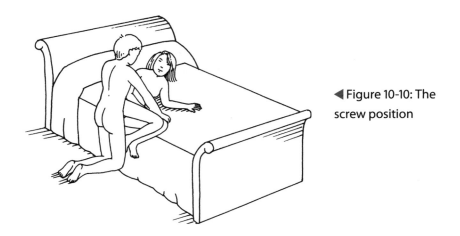

◀ Figure 10-10: The screw position

Lying Down Face-to-Face

Both people lie on their sides, facing each other, with their legs inter-crossed. Upside: intimate face-to-face contact. Downside: limited freedom of movement and thrusting ability. Note: This exact position is not in the Kama Sutra, but there is a similar pose called "Clasping Sideways" in which the lovers lie face-to-face fully stretched out against each other, with her legs open just enough for him to penetrate her.

Wheelbarrow

The wheelbarrow is a creative version of the standing rear entry. In this position, the woman leans toward the floor, and the man lifts her legs while she supports herself with her arms and hands. As you can probably guess from the name, this looks similar to an X-rated version of those old-fashioned wheelbarrow races that are a summer camp staple.

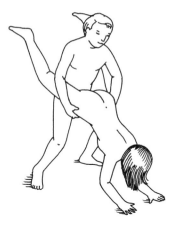

◀ Figure 10-11:
The wheelbarrow
position

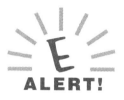

Some couples find the wheelbarrow position a little challenging. It can also be tricky if the woman is especially petite, or if there is a considerable height difference between the partners. In that case, it may help if the woman leans on a thick book or something else that will make her a bit taller.

Inverted Rear Entry

The inverted rear entry is a somewhat tricky position, and one that not everyone finds exciting. Both partners lie down on the bed, with the man underneath. The woman then lies on top of him, facing up, and the man enters her from underneath.

Kneeling with Woman Slightly on Top

A variation of the previously mentioned "sitting facing same direction" position involves the woman moving herself slightly up on the man, almost as if she's sitting in his lap, but remaining with her back to him. The man would have his legs folded underneath him. This is sometimes called the "Peas in a Pod" position.

Chapter 11

Advanced Positions

Let's face it, even your favorite tried-and-true position gets ho-hum after a while. To keep things exciting between the sheets, you need to constantly add new moves to your bedroom bag of tricks. Odds are, if you have been together for a while, you and your partner have already reached the "been there, done that" point when it comes to the basic positions, and possibly even a few of the more challenging ones. Master a few advanced maneuvers and you will get your sex life sizzling again.

Why Try New Positions?

They say variety is the spice of life, and variety is definitely the key to spicing up your love life. Boredom and predictability are the dual kiss of death for a hot sex life. Ancient Tantrics believed it was vital to bring consciousness into lovemaking. Therefore, they felt it was important to bring a lot of variety into the bedroom in order to keep the partners interested, focused on the moment, and in tune with their own body and that of their partner.

Tantrics also believed you should avoid the trap of falling into a rut, which is more likely to happen if you stick to an old faithful routine of the same two or three positions. By constantly mixing things up and trying new techniques, it is believed you put more thought into the activity.

More Esoteric Positions

You have already tried—and possibly even mastered—the basic standard positions outlined in Chapter 10. Now that you are ready to move on to something a little more unusual, you might want to give some of these more esoteric positions a try. These are not Kama Sutra positions. They are simply positions discovered by some really creative and adventurous people.

Amazon Position

In this position, the man lies flat on the bed and brings his knees up toward his chest. The woman then squats on top of him, lowering herself onto his penis. This can be a physically tiring position for the woman, and usually cannot be sustained for very long.

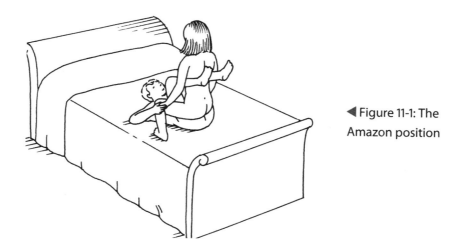

◀ Figure 11-1: The Amazon position

Twin Serpents

The woman lies on her back and the man lies on top of her, facing her feet. He enters her, and she can then wrap her legs up around his back to help maintain the position.

The Criss-Cross

This can also be thought of as a diagonal missionary position, or a sideway man-on-top. The woman lies flat on her back with the man above, positioned diagonally across her. Because the man is entering her on an angle, this can provide for new and interesting sensations. However, this position does not allow for a lot of thrusting or movement, and it can be challenging to maintain.

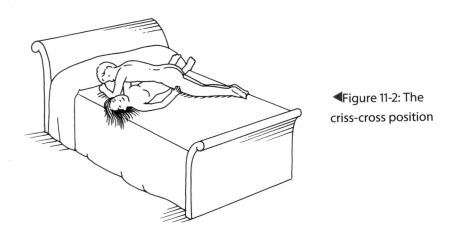

◀Figure 11-2: The
criss-cross position

Challenging Positions

If you are truly adventurous and/or experienced and have grown tired with all of the basic positions, and maybe even some of the advanced ones, you might want to try a few challenging maneuvers. Warning: These positions require strength and flexibility, and may prove difficult or impossible unless you are in great physical shape.

Backward Wheelbarrow

The man stands facing the woman. The woman wraps her legs around the man, gripping him with her thighs. She then leans backward, so her body is basically facing away from the man. She can support herself by placing her hands on the bed or floor. Essentially, she is upside-down doing a handstand away from the man. Needless to say, this requires considerable athletic ability on the woman's part and cannot be maintained for long because the blood will start rushing to her head (although some women claim that initially gives them quite a rush).

Acrobat Position

As the name implies, this is a challenging position requiring acrobatic-like flexibility on the woman's part. The man lies flat, and the woman lies on top of him, facing up. She mounts him, then tucks her feet underneath him and leans all the way back, so her upper body is resting on top of him. To picture this, imagine the woman is trying to do the limbo, with the bar very low. A bonus of this position: It acts as a great stretching maneuver.

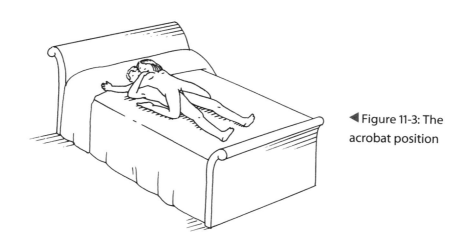

◀ Figure 11-3: The acrobat position

Armchair Position

This is another position that requires above-average upper arm strength on the part of the woman. The man lies on the bed, sitting up and supporting his weight with his hands. The woman then sits on top of him, leaning back with her feet resting on his shoulders. The man can lean back or forward more to adjust the thrust and angle.

Oral Sex Positions

Many people probably do not realize there are actually several different oral sex positions. Or perhaps they are just so happy to be getting oral sex that they don't really care what position it occurs in. Either way, you can make oral sex even more exciting by trying a few new positions.

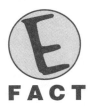

FACT

The standard (Burton) translation of the Kama Sutra outlines nine ways of performing fellatio, but says almost nothing about cunnilingus other than that the ways of kissing the yoni should be known by the ways of kissing the mouth. In general, though, the Kama Sutra considered oral sex to be morally improper.

Standing Fellatio

One of the most common oral sex positions, this is a basic position involving the man standing with the woman kneeling in front of him, facing him. She then performs oral sex on him while the man plays with her hair or simply enjoys the view. He might also gently guide her head into the correct position—he should never do this forcefully, and not at all if his partner does not like it.

Sitting Fellatio

If there is one thing better than fellatio, it is getting fellatio while sitting down. This is a real treat for the man—he gets pleasured while relaxing and not doing any work at all. The man sits on the edge of the bed or chair while the woman kneels in front of him. This is the position a couple uses when performing fellatio in unusual locations like at the movies (if you are very brave).

Woman on Top Cunnilingus

This is what you might consider the oral sex version of the cowgirl position. The man lies on his back, and the woman gets on top of him, with her genitals above his face. She can then lie back or forward. Women like this position because it allows them to be in control of the position and movement.

Man Kneeling Cunnilingus

This is probably the most common cunnilingus position. The woman lies on her back on a bed, so her waist is at the edge and her legs dangle over the side of the bed. The man then kneels in front of her. As he performs oral sex, the woman can lift her legs and wrap them around his neck or rest them on his shoulders.

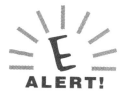

ALERT!

When it comes to trying new sexual positions, it is possible to be *too* adventurous. Sometimes a person will try to go through every position in the book in rapid succession. This quick and constant changing of position can be distracting and may in fact take away from the partner's pleasure because he or she doesn't get to stay in any one position long enough to enjoy it.

Sixty-Nine

The position known as "69" is probably the most well-known oral sex position. In this position, the partners lie on top of each other, facing each other, with one's head at the other's feet. Usually the woman is on top. They then align themselves so their mouths and genitals line up.

One-Sided Sixty-Nine

This position (also dubbed the "68" position) is similar to the 69, except the person on top is facing upward. As a result, only the person on top receives oral sex. This position offers the "giver" great access and the ability to more easily stimulate the receiver manually while giving oral sex.

Standing Sixty-Nine

This is an extremely challenging position—one which the vast majority of couples should not even attempt. Basically, it is only within the realm of possibility if one partner (presumably the man) is a weight lifter or otherwise has developed incredible upper body strength. The man stands and holds the woman in front of him upside down, so she is basically hanging there while they perform oral sex on each other.

Rear-Facing Woman on Top

In this position, the man is the one giving the oral sex. He lies on a bed, with his head hanging over the edge, and the woman stands next to the bed facing away from him, straddling his face. This can get tiring for the woman's legs, and may also give the man a headache. (The man should not lean his head too far over the bed, or the woman's weight could cause his neck to bend back at a dangerous angle.)

Anal Sex Positions

This probably goes without saying, but anal sex is not for everyone. While most men enjoy the sensation of engaging in anal sex as a "giver," some straight men worry that this gives off signals of homosexuality (which is not the case). For woman, anal sex can be uncomfortable, and often downright painful, especially if the man is well endowed.

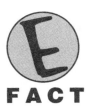

FACT

The most commonly used translations of the Kama Sutra (Burton's and Indra Sinha's) mention almost nothing about anal sex, except to say that it was practiced by people in certain parts of the country.

If you are going to attempt anal sex, be very sure to use lots of lubricant and make sure the woman is fully prepared. Start slowly. The man needs to exert a lot of self-control to resist the urge to launch into rapid thrusting right away. Instead, he needs to proceed slowly, inching in little by little with slow movement, until the woman feels comfortable to proceed more quickly.

Anal sex positions are often slight adaptations of "basic" sex positions—except of course for the fact that the penis enters the anus instead of the vagina.

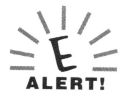

Never insert a penis (or anything else) into the vagina after it has been in the anus. This is an effective way to spread infections and bacteria. After anal sex, either wash the penis or put on a new condom before entering the vaginal area.

Rear Entry

The most popular anal sex position is very similar to the dog style position. The woman kneels on the bed or floor, with her rear end up in the air and her face downward. The man then kneels or stands behind her and enters her anally from behind. The one downside to this position is that the man often instinctively begins thrusting rapidly, as he would do with the dog style position. This can overwhelm the woman and may be painful.

Side-by-Side

Another anal variation of a basic position involves the couple lying in the spoon position, on their sides with the woman in front. The man then enters her from behind. The advantage of this position is that the woman can control the speed and intensity of the thrusting, which will probably make her more comfortable.

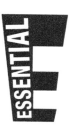

When first attempting anal sex, the man should start by stimulating the woman with his finger first. This will allow her to become accustomed to being penetrated there before being penetrated with the longer and wider penis. The greater freedom of movement with the finger allows the male to make the experience more pleasurable for the woman by moving his finger in various ways.

New Environments

You can also spice up your sex life not by changing the positions, but by changing the *place* in which you engage in those positions. Tantra encourages couples to stimulate their personal growth and push their boundaries by engaging in sex in a natural (outdoors) environment or in a new and exciting place.

Take It Outside

Many people find it thrilling to make love in the great outdoors. For one thing, outdoor settings like meadows, beaches, and mountains can be extremely romantic. They can also provide a sense of peace and calmness that help people relax. In addition, this type of scenery can provide a kind of cinematic backdrop—you almost feel as if you are acting out that sexy "making love on the beach scene" from your favorite movie. Unfortunately, for many people, this is not really a practical option. City dwellers could find this especially challenging. One option is to do some furtive fondling while discreetly covered up by a blanket in a semi-public location like the secluded area of a park. Even rural residents may not find the outdoors sex romp to be so easy—these days, even rural areas tend to have more than their share of passersby who could inadvertently interrupt your romantic romp. One option: If you have a pool or hot tub, trying engaging in sexual activities in or around these areas at night, when you won't be easily spotted.

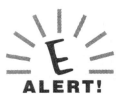

ALERT!

If you brave the great outdoors for sexual escapades, use some planning and precautions. Steer clear of areas where wild animals roam. And it is a good idea to lay down some blankets or towels to prevent sand, dirt, or other material from getting into the cracks and crevices of your body. And, needless to say, you should familiarize yourself with the characteristics of poison ivy plants.

You can also compromise by choosing a location that is outside but still very close to the house, such as a backyard hammock or the swing on your front porch. For increased privacy, a rooftop deck or second-story porch can offer the best of both worlds.

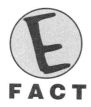

FACT

If you decide to engage in outdoor sex, you should keep in mind that very few exposed areas are completely "private" these days. Security cameras and other high-tech devices are almost everywhere, so it is possible that "eyes" (both the human and electronic variety) can easily be watching you, even if you think nobody is around.

On the Road

Many people find it exciting to engage in some illicit lovemaking while in a car. (Although some men find the idea of receiving fellatio while driving to be a turn-on, this is—needless to say—dangerous, and it is far wiser to pull off the road first.) This can bring back nostalgic memories of secret teenage backseat sex sessions. Some people, especially those with exhibitionist tendencies, find it arousing to have sex in a parking lot or in a roadside area, where passing motorists may spot a glimpse of them. However, this can be risky nowadays, so at the very least you should make sure the car doors are all locked, to make sure nobody could burst in on you unexpectedly.

A lot of people have also had exciting encounters in the back of a pickup truck, on a boat, or even astride a motorcycle, so don't be afraid to be creative.

All Around the House

Sometimes a change of scenery can be as simple as taking your tryst to a different part of the house. Most people have sex in the same exact room (usually their bedroom) every single time they make love. Boring! Think about the sexiest movies you have seen, where the hot-and-heavy "I've gotta have you *right now!*" scenes always take place in the kitchen, in the elevator, or maybe even at the office. Try heading into the kitchen—for added excitement, pretend you are at a dinner party and someone can burst into the kitchen at any minute. (Of course, if you are very brave, you could try this at a *real* dinner party where someone actually may burst in at any minute.) Or head to the couch and imagine you are two teenagers who could be caught by your parents at any moment.

If your living room has a fireplace, it can be very romantic to spread out a plush, cozy blanket and make love in front of the fire. For those with a home office, you can act out your "boss and secretary" role-playing fantasies in that room, while enjoying the added advantage of the benefits of office furniture, such as the wheeled leather office chair or the huge desk.

Position-Assisting Furniture

Need some help coming up with new and exciting positions? You are in luck—nowadays, there are lots of products available to help. Many companies are selling various types of lovemaking furniture, usually some type of wedge-shaped cushion or a futonlike piece of furniture.

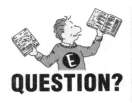

QUESTION?

Where can you buy this furniture?
You can find furniture, cushions, and related accessories at a variety of outlets, including adult shops and retail stores like Adam & Eve locations. If you prefer to shop online, there are many choices. Some suggestions to try: *www.loverocker.com* or *www.loving-angles.com.*

These furniture items are designed to be moved, flipped, turned, and otherwise manipulated to accommodate an assortment of sexual positions. What's more, they usually come with a manual or video demonstrating many positions—including, most likely, a few you hadn't thought of yet.

Positions for Conceiving

There are certain positions that are said to be more conducive to helping a couple conceive. Many experts feel that the missionary position (man on top) is the best position for those trying to conceive. Because this position allows for deeper penetration by the male, the theory is that the sperm will be closer to the cervix and stand a greater chance of reaching it in a timely manner. For additional help the woman can try elevating her hips with her hands or a pillow to allow her cervix to experience exposure to the maximum amount of semen. (The theory here being that in this position less semen will drip out prematurely.)

But for those who don't like the missionary position or get bored with it, there are other positions that can foster good baby-making environments. These generally include the rear-entry positions, lying side-by-side, and other postures that encourage deep penetration. Some clinicians also state that the woman lying in bed (again on her back with her hips elevated by a pillow) for up to a half-hour after sex can increase the chances of successful conception. A woman's OB/GYN may be able to offer some helpful advice with regard to this topic.

In addition the positions that are considered the worst for conception are any of the woman-on-top positions and any standing or sitting positions, as these positions have gravity working against the flow of sperm.

Taking it a step further, some people believe that certain positions are also more conducive to allowing a couple to conceive a baby of specific *gender*, but there is no scientific proof that a certain position determines the baby's gender. Some old wives' tales on this subject include using the rear-entry or standing positions to guarantee a boy and using the missionary and woman on top to ensure a girl. Of course, these are only superstitions, but if you want to give these myths a try, feel free—there's no harm in trying, and practicing can be wonderful.

Positions During Pregnancy

Suppose you have already conceived (in whatever position worked for you). Congratulations! This is an exciting time, but—as any couple that has ever been expecting can attest—it is also a time fraught with lots of things to worry about. Somewhere in those many worries may be the effects the pregnancy may have on your sex life. Among other things, you may now be wondering about the best—or safest—sexual positions for a pregnant woman. It is a good idea to consult with your doctor, especially if you have any medical complications or have a high-risk pregnancy. But in general, most women are able to sustain a normal, healthy sex life well into their pregnancy. As the pregnancy progresses, however, the woman may feel the need to avoid deep thrusting. Obviously, it's a good idea to avoid positions where the man's weight is on her belly, especially later in pregnancy.

Some popular positions during pregnancy include lying side by side in the spoon position, woman on top, and sitting positions, all of which put no extra weight on the uterus and allow the woman to control the depth of the penetration to where she is comfortable. Also use the bed as a prop whenever possible to take some of the weight off the woman and also as a way to prop her up into comfortable positions.

Chapter 12

Rituals and Ceremonies

The concept of a ritual or ceremony may invoke thoughts of formality and seriousness, but that is not necessarily the case at all. In fact, when it comes to romantic rituals, fun and spontaneity are often the primary goals. While there are numerous books and other resources that can give you ideas for enjoyable rituals, it will probably be more fun and meaningful for you to develop your own loving rituals. A ritual can be any kind of event, routine, or tradition that makes you feel sexy and more connected to your partner.

Personal Rituals

Rituals can also have special and personal sentimental significance. If your partner gave you a beautiful bouquet of red roses on your first date, you may create a ritual in which you spread rose petals out around your sacred sex area before a romantic evening.

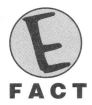

FACT

A ritual can be as simple as lighting your partner's favorite scent of candles for your traditional Saturday night rendezvous. Or it could even be booking "your" table at your favorite romantic restaurant.

Or maybe your ritual will be something a bit racier, like taking turns performing striptease dances for each other. Some couples like to watch a movie (be it a romantic film or an X-rated flick) as a ritual to get them in the mood for sex.

If you are the creative types, you could take turns writing poems and reading them to each other, or singing a song you wrote especially for your partner.

The ritual itself is not as important as the thought behind it, and the fact that you have created this special event together, something you find mutually exciting that you can share on special occasions.

You probably would not want to engage in the same ritual every time you make love, or the novelty will wear off quickly and things will get boring. On the other hand, a familiar ritual can sometimes be comforting, making you feel more at ease.

Tantric Rituals

In its ancient form, Tantra revolved around rituals, and lots of them. Everything of importance was done in a ritualistic manner, and the sacred rituals were viewed with utmost respect and reverence. While the most controversial and high profile of these rituals involves sex, Tantrics observed rituals of many types, for lots of different purposes. There were rituals for relieving stress, other rituals for promoting spirituality, and still more rituals for sexual healing and connecting emotionally with one's partner.

Rituals in Tantric History

Rituals of many types have been a central part of Tantric traditions since the very beginning. Most of the common ancient rituals are as old as Tantra itself. In fact, in the early days, this was one of the things Tantra was most famous for. Tantric rituals—especially those involving sex—were a classic hallmark of Tantric practices.

Taoism and Tantra

Rituals were central themes of both Tantra and Taoism in ancient times. These rituals were designed to take the act of lovemaking and transport it to a whole new level—thus elevating the routine sexual union to a higher spiritual plane. Both Taoism and Tantra viewed sexual rituals as the most effective way to transcend physical ecstasy and enter spiritual bliss.

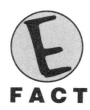

FACT

Virtually every traditional Taoist ritual involved a *jiao*. This was a ritual offering or routine. It was done with a specific goal in mind—for example, to request fruitful crops or seek eternal peace for the soul of someone who recently died.

The Tantric rituals have mainly managed to survive only thanks to the hard work of a few dedicated gurus and yogis in the east, who have carefully recorded, preserved, and passed down these rituals so their importance can live on through future generations.

Ancient Tantric sexual rituals often included many instantly recognizable Tantric hallmarks: chanting and meditation as well as sensual delights such as candles and music, wine, etc.

The Lost Rituals

Unfortunately, some sexual rites practiced by ancient Tantrics are no longer documented in modern texts. Perhaps because they were misunderstood during various periods in history, these acts were often practiced in secret and kept "underground," remaining both mysterious and magical. People who participated in these rituals were typically sworn to secrecy, and never spoke of the rituals outside of their closed circle, so the specific activities involved in these rituals remained a mystery to everyone except those who had witnessed the events firsthand. The details were passed down almost completely by word of mouth, and many were lost along the way. These rituals were considered so powerful that they were only revealed to a select few. Unless someone was advanced along the spiritual path, they weren't considered ready to partake in such rituals, as it was believed they would get lost in the purely sexual aspects and forget their spiritual purpose.

And then there are other rituals that are deemed too complicated, especially when translated from Tantric texts, to be easily understood by westerners.

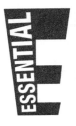

Most Tantric rituals had some common central traits, including the use of sacred objects. Great importance was placed upon these items, which include some of the symbols and items mentioned in Chapter 2. For example, the vajra and bell are both frequently part of Tantric rituals, as is the *phurpa* (a magic dagger believed to help conquer bad spirits).

Sex Rituals

As you have probably realized by now, Tantrics (like everyone else) practiced rituals of many kinds, including many that were totally innocent and not related to sex in any way. These other rituals may have involved yoga, meditation, chanting, and many other activities that were not controversial in any way. But it is the sexual rituals that have gained the most notoriety and attention. Not surprisingly, these are the rituals that most people are generally the most curious about, and the ones they always immediately associate with Tantra.

It is important to note that to Tantrics, these sexual rituals were much more than just a good time. While it is true that in some cases they may have resembled orgies from outside appearances, they had a much deeper purpose to the people who practiced them. These rituals were seen as a means to an end—the end being the sought-after state of higher consciousness. Participants in sexual rituals were seeking spiritual liberation and wanted to achieve a oneness with the universe. This was their traditional way of pursuing that goal.

Still, there are those Tantric gurus and experts who claim that the ritualistic sexual exploits of ancient Tantrics have been greatly exaggerated or misunderstood. Although many ancient Hindu texts give elaborate directions and descriptions of group sexual rituals, these gurus say these writing were not meant to be taken literally. In their opinion, the passages were meant symbolically, or were translated incorrectly or taken out of context. However, there seems to be ample proof that ritualized sex activities did play a role in Tantric practices.

Modern Western Rituals

Rituals are certainly not unique to Tantra. Almost every society of people (from all regions of the world) has its own group of rituals. Neither are rituals purely a thing of the past. Many people practice rituals, even if they do not consciously acknowledge them as such.

Even here in the West, among mainstream society, people have their fair share of rituals—including both romantic and sexual rituals—although they do not always view these practices as rituals, per se. For example, there is the popular Valentine's Day tradition of going to a fancy restaurant for a nice romantic dinner. Likewise, for many couples there is a special dinner or other event to mark the wedding anniversary. And many people arrange a special setting in advance for the first time they expect to have sex with their partner.

Couples often develop their own unique romantic rituals as well. For example, they may develop a routine of having a romantic sexual tryst every Saturday night, following a night of dinner and dancing.

Sex Rituals in Other Religions

While a core part of Taoist and Tantric traditions, sex-related rituals certainly were not limited to only the followers of these philosophies, by any means. Paganism recognized the importance of sexual rites and rituals, and the power that could be derived from the sex act.

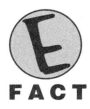

FACT

In ancient times, pagan rituals had a strong focus on sex. Many common pagan rituals involved participants having sex with others besides their partners. Today, some modern-day Wiccans practice a ritual called the Great Rite, which involves the union (sometimes symbolic as opposed to physical) between two people.

It is believed that other religions and belief systems also practiced sexual rituals, but have "watered down" that part of their histories by referring to these acts in ambiguous, abstract terms. They may have devised innocent-sounding euphemisms for these rituals, or buried them in harmless folklore or entertaining stories. You would need to try and read between the lines and guess at what the story might be suggesting. Unless you knew the true meaning behind the stories, it would be tough to guess their more explicit origins.

The Da Vinci Code Effect

Sex rituals have become a hot topic of discussion lately, in great part because of Dan Brown's blockbuster novel *The Da Vinci Code*. As part of the book's central plot, the author describes ceremonial practices involving sexual activities. He goes into great detail in depicting the rituals, the activities involved, and the significance these rituals held in relation to the religious and spiritual beliefs of the participants.

However, this aspect of the book was met with a loud (and harsh) backlash. In the novel, the narrator refers to a sexual initiation rite as a common part of early Christianity. He further states that these rituals were a standard and accepted practice in early Christian and Jewish worship. Critics have reacted strongly, pointing out that—despite what is depicted in the novel—there is no proof that early Christians or Jewish people engaged in these rituals.

Unlike in Taoism or Tantra, where sex and rituals are often connected in various ways, Christian and Jewish texts and teachings contain no mention of ritualized sex. In fact, these two religions make little or no connection between sex and worship at all.

It would have seemed more plausible if Dan Brown had attributed these activities to Tantric or Tao practitioners—but of course that would not have fit with his central plot, that Christ had a secret lineage originating from a child born as a result of his relationship with Mary Magdalene. In order to work the sex rituals into the plot, Brown needed to connect them to the Christian religion, which is central to the book.

Needless to say, this aspect of the novel also generated a strong negative reaction from church leaders and religious groups.

The Basics of Rituals

People of all faiths, nationalities, and belief systems practice rituals of many types, and for many reasons. There are rituals surrounding holidays, religious events, family traditions, and many other types of rituals. Many of these are innocuous and innocent. Often we do them without even thinking about them. The downside, of course, is that we find ourselves automatically going through the motions, carrying out our rituals without even giving a thought as to the meaning or tradition behind them.

Common Theme of Rituals

A ritual act is basically a rite or process with a definite intention or goal. It has some routine, repetitive acts to it, and perhaps a specific timeline or sequence of events that must be followed. Although usually planned, rituals can also be practiced spontaneously. Perhaps most importantly, a ritual usually has some kind of deeper meaner, possibly a spiritual or psychological purpose. It often carries a lot of symbolism.

The Importance of Rituals

Rituals of all types are important to people for many reasons. First, there is the aspect of honoring tradition. There can be powerful sentimental value in knowing you are carrying on the same traditional rituals practiced by people before you.

Rituals are also by definition routine, which translates to safety, predictability, and familiarity, all of which can be soothing, especially in times of stress. There is something comforting about knowing what will happen and being able to count on the sequence of events.

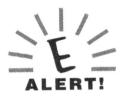

ALERT!

While rituals can provide a comforting sense of security and routine, one should avoid becoming too dependent on a lot of rituals. This can quickly take the form of falling into a rut, and can also prevent a person from acting spontaneously. In other words, rituals should not interfere with one's ability to do other things that might be enjoyed.

Rituals can also bring people together. A group of people who practice a common ritual (whether together or individually) share a positive bonding experience. This can bring people together and foster strong connections.

The Basic Secret Rite

While there were many types of sexual rituals practiced by Tantrics over the years, the most basic and probably the most easily understood is the secret rite, or the basic sexual ritual, also known as *Maithuna Sadhana* in Tantra. Although this is a simplified description, here is a basic overview of how this ritual might go.

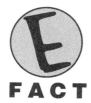

FACT

Maithuna is a Sanskrit term for "union," which is often used to refer to a sexual union. It represents a spiritual unification for the purpose of creating spiritual balance and harmony. Maithuna Sadhana is the spiritual (and often physical) union and oneness of man and woman.

The Warm-Up Stage

Before starting the ritual itself, the proper setting must be established by the careful placement of candles, the selection of music, and the lighting of a fire.

When the time is right, the couple begins the ritual by taking a bath or shower. They then massage each other with oils. Often, they then engage in a period of stretching, yoga, or even dancing, in order to relax the muscles and to get them in the proper frame of mind.

Then they sit closely together and do some simple meditation routines. Along the way, they focus on their breathing, trying to synchronize their breathing patterns.

Honoring Each Other

At this point, they move on to the main part of the ritual: honoring each other. Traditionally, the woman is honored first. Her partner begins worshipping her as a goddess, adorning her with beautiful scarves and fabrics and massaging her with oil. He then slowly and gradually begins touching her body in a very deliberate and predetermined sequence. Meanwhile, his partner visualizes techniques to imagine her energy force growing increasingly stronger and rising up through her body.

The man takes occasional breaks to meditate, during which time he might gaze into the fire or candle. During this process, the man (and possibly the woman) recite certain chants and mantras. For the man, these repetitive mantras often include telling the woman how beautiful she is, and how much he worships her as his goddess.

The couple then shifts roles, with the woman worshipping her partner.

Lovemaking Takes Place

When worship is finished, the couple begins the actual act of lovemaking. In ancient texts, the woman is almost always described as sitting on the right side of the man when the ritual begins, and then moves to his left side for this stage of actual lovemaking.

While the specific positions can vary, the sequence is often discussed and agreed upon beforehand. If the couple has a specific purpose in mind, a goal they wish to achieve through this ritual—conceiving a child, for example, or attaining sexual healing—they would constantly visualize it throughout this part of the ritual.

If the man ejaculates, the couple remains in union for as long as possible afterward, allowing the woman to absorb his vital life energy.

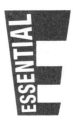

As part of the preparations for the ritual, the couple should have a bowl or tray of fruits or other treats waiting nearby for when they have finished making love. Ancient Tantric practitioners considered this important, as the process was believed to be draining, and often worked up hunger and thirst. It was viewed as important that the couple be able to replenish their energy following the sexual union.

The sexual ritual was often conducted on specific days of the month, commonly on "desirable" times during the woman's menstrual cycle.

The Rite of the Five Essentials

A ritual practiced by Tantrics in India, the Rite of the Five Essentials was one of the most well-known ritual traditions. It was sometimes also known as the Tantric Eucharist or the Ritual of the Five M's.

The Five Essential Elements

As you can probably guess from its name, traditionally this ritual consisted of five main essential elements. Those were: meat, fish, wine, grains, and sexual union. These were symbolic of the essential ingredients of the higher universe, and also corresponded to the five elements of earth (water, fire, air, space, and earth).

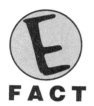

FACT

Traditionally, ritual lovemaking events incorporated indulgences for all of the senses. Tantrics believed it was important to experience all of the sensual pleasures, because it was believed that spiritual liberation could only be achieved once all of the physical desires were satisfied.

The Ritual Proceeds

This ritual generally took place at night, almost always near an open fire, which was considered an essential element. Color was also important—generally, red played a major role because it was believed to stimulate the male sexual energies. The woman would be anointed with five essential oils.

After going through all the usual preparatory steps like burning incense and enjoying some music, they would proceed to the five-step part of the ritual. They would start by enjoying the wine. They then would consume the meat, followed by the fish. They then shared the grains. At this point, the couple would proceed to passionate lovemaking.

This ritual was considered most powerful and effective when each of the five elements was viewed as symbolizing a higher purpose or goal.

Chakra Puja

The Chakra Puja (literally translated as "circle worship") is one of the oldest practices of traditional Tantra. Also known as "group worship," this ritual—and the similar ritual of Vasishtha—involved up to eight couples. The general goal of this ritual is a group effort in pursuit of higher consciousness.

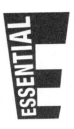

In some ancient Tantric rituals, menstrual fluid played an important role. Far from being reviled, this fluid was generally revered. It was seen as mystical and magical, because of its power to create life. In some rituals, this fluid was used in worship. Along the same lines, a menstruating woman was also often given a special place of honor.

Like many ancient Tantric sex rituals, especially those involving large groups of people, the preparations and trappings of this event were elaborate. The participants would often start out by enjoying wine and perhaps some cannabis. This ritual would often include a lengthy assortment of Tantric techniques, including meditation, mantras, yantras, purification, body worship, and other techniques. The Tantric couples would sit in a circle and take turns actively participating in various practices, including sexual unions. According to some descriptions, male and female partners would be assigned at random. Other reports describe the guru assigning participants a partner of the opposite sex. Many accounts describe the guru or leader kicking off the action by having sex with a nude young woman while the others watched.

Chapter 13

Chakras

It would be impossible to discuss Tantra without mentioning chakras. Chakras are an important part of your spiritual growth through Tantric teachings. They represent the energy of life, the power sources that keep your physical, emotional, and spiritual systems running properly. If the chakras become clogged or stop working properly, they cannot pump or circulate our energies as they should. By learning about your chakras and how they work, you can help alleviate problems that may be causing your energy sources to become "clogged."

Origins of Chakras

The concept of chakras, while not believed to date back to the very beginning of Tantra, have now become an integral part of the Tantric philosophy. Chakras are the spiritual energy centers, or cores, that are present in every body. Although some gurus were said to be able to actually see the chakras, they are generally regarded as a symbolic entity, like an aura. Think of them as spiritual fields, each of which is associated with special traits and characteristics. The chakras run directly down the center of the body, located along the backbone, and correspond to parts of the endocrine system and nervous system.

Chakras and Their Roots

It is believed that the idea of chakras may have originated from the concept of a vital force (known as a *prana*) that was described in the earliest Upanishads (sacred written texts) dating back to eighth century B.C. But it wasn't until a few hundred years later that chakras were specifically mentioned in the sacred texts. Throughout the years, the chakras (in various forms) were mentioned in many different texts and published works.

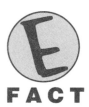

FACT

The word *chakra* is Sanskrit for "wheel" or "disk." The wheel is also symbolic for the sun, which is of course the most powerful energy source in the universe. Sometimes the term *chakra* is also used to mean a gathering of Tantrics.

As Tantra evolved into more modern incarnations, the chakras were accentuated by specific colors, element symbols, and other characteristics that were assigned to each chakra. As a result, later texts provide much more detailed and intricate descriptions of chakras, including shapes, colors, number of petals found on the lotus representing each chakra, etc. However, many Tantra gurus advise students to focus on the main elements of each chakra, to avoid getting distracted or overwhelmed by all of the minute details.

Chakras in Written Texts

Chakras have been described in many accounts appearing in modern Western literature. Many of these references were in works by Charles W. Leadbeater, who in the late 1800s became one of the founding members of the Theosophical Society. Leadbeater was most famous for his claims of being a clairvoyant and having occult powers.

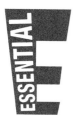

Charles W. Leadbeater received notoriety for accusations that he had improper sexual contact with some of his young students. He claimed that he was simply explaining the practice of masturbation to boys so they would understand the topic and not feel shame if they engaged in masturbation. Leadbeater died without ever being charged with any illegal offense.

Leadbeater wrote about the chakras in great detail in the early twentieth century. Several other authors from around the same time also covered the topic in detail, often by commissioning translations of early Hindu texts. Unfortunately, it is believed that somehow much of the original points got "lost in translation." As a result, many people believe the modern description of chakras differ greatly from the way they were originally depicted in ancient texts. For one thing, the earliest texts reportedly only referred to four main chakras: those at the heart, throat, head, and navel. (The chakras that fall below the waist were viewed as more of a physical entity than a spiritual force, so they were grouped into a special, separate category.)

Understanding Chakras

By studying the chakras and what they mean, it is believed you can make positive changes in your life. The concept of chakras is rooted in the mind-body connection—or, more accurately, the spirit/body connection. If you feel pain or illness in a certain part of your body, the cause may be rooted in the corresponding chakra. Once you learn to evaluate and "diagnose" your chakras, you can see where your energy forces are lagging, figure out what is causing the problem, and (most important) fix it.

Each chakra symbolizes one aspect of our spiritual being, our state of consciousness. By improving the state of our chakras, we can achieve spiritual balance and attain a higher state of consciousness. And, of course, one of the main goals of Tantra is to continually pursue a higher state of consciousness, on the quest to become a more enlightened being and grow closer to the higher power.

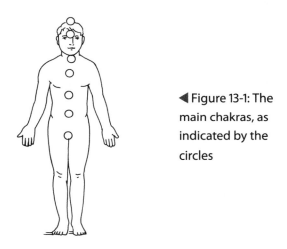

◀ Figure 13-1: The main chakras, as indicated by the circles

There are seven main chakras in Hindu Tantra: sahasrara, ajna, vishuddha, anahata, manipura, swadhisthana, and muladhara.

Sahasrara

Sahasrara is known as "the crown chakra." As you can probably guess from that nickname, it is located at the top of the head. A fitting location, since this chakra is believed to be the superior chakra, which is above all of the others. This represents a person or being who is immortal or godlike. It can also represent your connection with God, the universe, or a higher power. It is believed that when your energy force builds up and reaches your crown chakra, you will feel an unparalleled connection with the universe and the world around you.

The crown chakra corresponds with the pituitary gland, which controls the other parts of the endocrine system. This is represented by white, symbolizing a Godlike higher power and light. It is believed that if this chakra is closed, you will be unable to transcend your sacred sex into a spiritual experience. However, if it is open, you will be able to turn sexual union into a mystical experience.

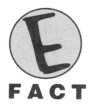

FACT

The chakras are also sometimes referred to as "the Tree of Life." Tantrics use the analogy that all parts of the tree serve an important and necessary function: You cannot have the fruit without the limbs; you cannot have the trunk without the roots, etc. Each chakra is believed to be equally valuable and important.

Ajna

Ajna, known as "the third eye," is the chakra that represents self-discovery, intuition, and enlightenment. Its color is indigo. This corresponds to the pineal gland, which is responsible for the production of melatonin, a hormone that regulates our sleep cycles. It is fitting then that this chakra is often symbolically associated with a spiritual "awakening." The third eye is also associated with intuition and psychic sensitivity, traits believed to be more powerful in women.

Vishuddha

Vishuddha is the chakra located at the base of the throat and symbolizes verbalization, or saying what needs to be said. It is related to communication and self-expression. If this chakra is under active, you may be timid or avoid speaking up for yourself. As a result, you may end up simply going along with your partner's wishes. If it is overactive, you will be the kind of person who never shuts up. This chakra is considered important for good communication and expressing one's thoughts and feelings. It corresponds with the thyroid gland, responsible for weight, growth, and maturity. Its color is blue.

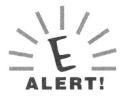

ALERT!

Each chakra is associated with a specific organ or group of organs. Tantrics believe that many health problems can be traced to an imbalance or weakness in the corresponding chakras. Thus, by ensuring your chakras are open and well-balanced, you can spare yourself considerable health problems.

Anahata

Anahata is located in the chest, near the heart, so it is not surprising that it symbolizes love and happiness, joy and laughter. When you lose a love, you are said to be heartbroken. Sometimes you may feel actually pain or tightness in your chest, which can be connected to this chakra. It corresponds with the thymus gland, which affects the immune system. Naturally, it is also connected to the heart and circulatory system. If this chakra is underactive, you are short on compassion and kindness. If it is overactive, you are overly affectionate and may smother people with affection. Its color is green, symbolizing growth. Jealousy can also be associated with an unbalanced anahata. (Perhaps this is where the term "green-eyed monster" comes from.)

Manipura

Manipura is the chakra located in the abdomen, below the rib cage. It is associated with feelings of control and anger. Self-esteem and the ego are also associated with this chakra. It corresponds with the pancreas, which controls the breakdown of sugar and is connected to diabetes. If this chakra is low on energy, you feel submissive, nervous, and self-conscious. (Fittingly, you may feel like you have "butterflies in your stomach.") If this chakra has too much energy, you will be bossy and controlling. This chakra is designated by the color yellow, symbolizing a sunny disposition and radiance.

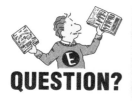

QUESTION?

What is chakra visulation?

Chakra visualization is a common practice incorporated into meditation rituals. To do this, you stimulate each chakra individually by focusing your energy on each particular energy center for several minutes, one at a time. As you do this, visualize a bright light in the color corresponding to that chakra. Conclude by imagining a bright light flowing through all the chakras.

Swadhisthana

Swadhisthana is located between the navel and the groin area. It is associated with the qualities of emotion and sexuality. This chakra is also connected to the idea of family and procreation. It corresponds with the reproductive organs (ovaries or testes) where sex hormones are created. It is also seen as the body's center of gravity. Fitness professionals often refer to this area as the body's core. If this chakra is low on energy, you may feel cold or distant toward other people and have trouble forming emotional bonds. However, if it has too much energy, you will get overly emotional and perhaps clingy or possessive. Its color is orange, and it is associated with the water element.

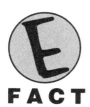

FACT

Because they are based on spiritual concepts, the role of chakras cannot be proven or addressed by the modern medical community. Needless to say, this provides skeptics with plenty of ammunition. However, many people in the medical field have acknowledged the mind-body connection, and the spirit/body connection of the chakras works in a similar manner.

Muladhara

Muladhara is the base chakra. It is located in the genital region, often said to be at the perineum, near the anal area. Because it is near the location of childbirth, the base chakra is often equated with life. This chakra also represents survival and the things needed for basic survival. If you are insecure about your job and ability to support yourself, this may cause problems with the base chakra. The Muladhara chakra is believed to correspond with the adrenal gland. Of course, it is the adrenal gland (and adrenaline) that comes into play in situations where we are in danger or must fight to survive. This chakra—which represents the basic concept of security and survival—is assigned a red color, and it is associated with the earth element. If this chakra has too little energy, you may feel insecure or nervous. You may also have negative feelings associated with sex. If it has too much energy, you will have a tendency to be too sure of yourself, acting overconfident and materialistic.

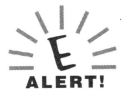

ALERT!

Because the chakras are all connected, they can each affect the others. A problem with one chakra will often cause a ripple effect that will throw the other chakras out of whack. If several of your chakras do not seem right, you may need to do some investigating to figure out which one initially caused the problem.

Chakras and Energy

As stated earlier, chakras are based on the concept of the wheel. That is because the chakra is a core of energy that then radiates out to the other parts of the body. Picture a magnetic field emanating from its source. When there is tension or pain in a particular part of your spirit or consciousness, it will affect your energy flow and will be reflected by pain in the areas of your corresponding chakras.

Tantrics believe that by channeling sexual energy and your life force up and down the inner flute into the chakras, you will be able to destroy the physical, mental, and emotional roadblocks that are standing in the way of your spiritual bliss.

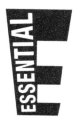

The inner flute—also called "the hollow bamboo"—is often envisioned as a channel that connects the genitals to the brain. Think of it as a train, with the chakras being on an axis that serves as the train tracks. By keeping all of your chakras in an open and receptive state, you give positive energy an easy passage through the inner flute.

Opening Chakras

If your chakras are out of whack, don't despair. You can take certain steps to help open the chakras, allowing them to better regulate the flow of energy. One way to open chakras is by employing mudras, the sacred Tantra hand movements and gestures. You sit in a comfortable position (traditionally, in the cross-legged yoga position). Then you move your hands and fingers into the proper mudra position corresponding to the specific chakras on which you want to focus. At the same time, you should alternate between chanting and meditating.

You can also open and stimulate the chakras by doing a chakra massage. This is a good technique for a couple to perform together, taking turns doing a chakra massage on each other. Have your partner lie down on her or his back (naked, preferably). You then start at the lowest chakra, massaging it for several minutes, and then working your way up, spending roughly the same amount of time on each chakra.

Tibetan Chakras

The chakras previously described are related to Hindu Tantra. Tibetan Tantra recognizes a different set of chakras—consisting of a variable number from four to ten. As explained earlier, the sahasrara (located at the top of the head) is considered the most important chakra in Hindu Tantra, symbolizing the highest state of consciousness. The opposite is true with Tibetan chakras: The root chakra is at the top of the head, and you progress downward toward the heart for higher states of consciousness.

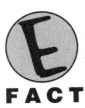

FACT

In addition to chakras recognized by Hindu Tantra and Tibetan Tantra, there are also chakras observed by other religions and philosophies. In Peru, the Q'ero tribe recognizes nine chakras, while certain Native American tribes believe the lowest chakra is actually at the very tip of the genitals.

Influencing Chakras

So what do you do if there is a problem or imbalance with your chakras? You need to try to influence them and make adjustments to their status so they can begin absorbing and processing energy properly. This can be done in a variety of ways. First, you can employ the mudras techniques described previously. In addition, you can use a combination of chanting and meditation. Certain types of massage and reflexology are also said to be helpful in influencing your chakras. Yoga is thought to be very useful in adjusting your chakras as well. You can even buy types of crystals that will supposedly help influence the chakras.

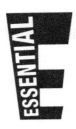

ESSENTIAL

It is believed that you can affect your chakras by eating specific types of foods. For example, eating root vegetables like carrots and beets can help your muladhara (the root chakra), while dairy foods and pasta are thought to be good for your manipura.

Getting Your Chakras in Sync as a Couple

For two people in a romantic relationship, it is important that their chakras be in harmony. If this is not the case, it will cause tensions and problems between them. The chakras of the two genders tend to complement each other, fitting together nicely like puzzle pieces. So, if a chakra is inverted on the man, it tends to be outward-facing on the woman, and vice versa. The most obvious example of this is the chakra located in the groin area. Needless to say, this part of the body on a man sticks out, while this area of a woman is inverted like a valley.

In Tantra, it is considered very important for a couple to get their chakras in sync for a happy, harmonious union. People should also strive to achieve a positive energy state for their chakras, which will then supposedly attract their partner with a magnetic-like energy field.

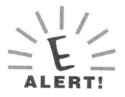

Want to evaluate the current status of your chakras? The Web site Eclectic Energies (*www.eclecticenergies.com*) offers a handy little self-test for just this purpose. It is a comprehensive test consisting of fifty-six questions, so it may take a little time, but at the end you will have a helpful analysis of the state of your chakras.

Chakra Spooning

Somraj Pokras is the founder of Tantra at Tahoe and the author of numerous e-books and online courses related to Tantra. He recommends this exercise—which he calls "Chakra Spooning"—to help synchronize your chakras with your partner's. This is also a great way to sustain your spiritual energies after lovemaking.

1. Lie down on something soft and comfortable.
2. Spoon. This means lying on your sides, one in front of the other, in a close embrace. (Most couples generally spoon with the same partner in front every time, but it can be fun to switch this up once in a while.)
3. The person in back places his or her hand on the other's first chakra.
4. The person in the inner position sets the breathing pattern by doing deep, slow belly breathing. The partner should follow this rhythm.
5. Together, both of you should visualize your breath drawing energy into your first chakras and swirling together. Imagine the energy releasing as you exhale.

6. Breathe into each chakra at least three times. If it seems like a particular chakra needs more attention, give it as many additional breaths as you feel necessary.
7. When ready, the inside person moves on to the second chakra, and the partner follows.
8. After breathing into the last chakra, lie together quietly and feel the energies in your bodies. Discuss your feelings and experiences with each other.

Chapter 14

The Tantric Way of Life

Once you seriously delve into it, Tantra is not something you can simply turn on and off when it is convenient for you. It becomes a part of you, your life, and everything you do. Whether you consciously realize it or not, Tantra will spill over into every part of your life and touch everything and everyone around you. There really is no such thing as a "part-time Tantric." It is something you will benefit from every hour of every day. Tantra truly is a total way of life.

Bring Tantra into Your Entire Life

If you are adopting Tantra as a new spiritual direction, you probably already expect it to have major ramifications for your entire life overall. That is to be anticipated—and welcomed, since the results are almost sure to be an improvement. It would be silly not to expect this vast body of knowledge and the spiritual awakening that it creates to touch every part of your world.

But if you plan to study Tantra in limited quantities, only to improve certain areas of your life such as your sexual relations, you may not realize the far-reaching effects this newfound knowledge will have on the rest of your world. Remember, *Tantra* is based on a word meaning "to weave," so it is perhaps fitting that the Tantric attitudes will soon weave their way into every facet of your life, making positive changes in your entire world.

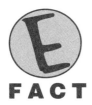

FACT

It may sound cliché, but Tantra truly believes in the importance of each person making a difference in the world. This should be your ultimate goal. Strive to bring greater meaning to your existence, to fulfill your destiny and make a positive contribution to the universe. Never stop seeking the deeper meaning of your life and your place in the world.

You will begin to look at the universe in a new and wondrous way. You will act differently and interact differently with people around you and the environment as a whole. You will have new appreciation and respect for your world, and you will achieve states of bliss and contentment that may take you by surprise.

Make Active Changes

This transformation is bound to happen, whether you realize it or not—and regardless of whether you make any conscious effort on your part. But if you are wise, you will not just sit back and wait for this inevitable occurrence—you will be proactive, and help it happen. Actively seek out opportunities to see the world in new and different ways. Embrace things that bring peace and harmony to your world. Take time to notice and appreciate the universe around you, and all the little things that bring bliss into your life.

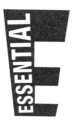

While many Tantric techniques stress control in various forms, you should have the clarity to realize that you will not always have control over your situation or your feelings. Accept this, and work with it. If you are angry or frustrated, channel that energy for a vigorous yoga work-out or even an intense session of passionate lovemaking.

Appreciate Things Around You

Tantra teaches the importance of focus and clarity. When you reduce the stress in your life and use meditation and other techniques to help yourself focus more clearly, you start seeing and appreciating things you barely noticed before.

Spend as much time outdoors as possible, to enjoy a union with nature and the universe around you. Take notice of all of the wondrous things in nature, many of which can serve as examples for your own life. For example, a tree can stand mighty and tall, but it once started out as a very tiny seedling. It was only through the help of fertile soil and the nourishment of nature that the tree was able to thrive and grow. In a similar way, people can only thrive and grow if they receive proper nourishment (both physical and spiritual) and assistance.

Make Tantra a Way of Life

You should strive to incorporate Tantra and the Tantric principles into your entire world and all aspects of your life. Don't worry: This will be a good thing, and something you will enjoy doing. The positive energy and spiritual contentment you achieve through Tantra is bound to have a positive impact on every part of your life.

The Benefits of a Tantric Lifestyle

It is impossible to count all the benefits you will reap from incorporating Tantra into everything you do and making its beliefs a way of life. Simply put, it will change everything—for the better.

Tantrics believe that when you adopt Tantra as a way of life, you open yourself up to experiencing more bliss, joy, peace, and harmony than you would have ever thought possible. You will have more inner peace, enjoy a balanced life, and greatly enhance your relationships with those around you. You will greatly reduce or eliminate much of the stress from your life, and you will learn effective techniques for dealing with the stress you cannot avoid.

Your relationships with loved ones (especially your spouse or partner) will blossom, and your interactions with every person you come in contact with will also improve.

Make It Happen

So how do you do this, exactly? By making a conscious effort to bring all of the basic philosophies of Tantra into every area of your life. You should not just discuss Tantra or simply study it; you should embody it. Make it such a part of your life that it takes over automatically and you act in Tantric ways without even giving it a second thought. In other words, don't just talk the talk—you also need to walk the walk.

As soon as you wake in the morning, take time to appreciate your life and be thankful for another day. Show gratitude to the universe for all of your blessings, and resolve to make the day ahead of you count. Devote some time to meditation and deep breathing, so you can embark on your day with a calm attitude and clear mind.

Make a mental plan for your day, and decide how you will make a positive contribution to the universe and to the lives of people around you.

Take time to appreciate all of the things around you, especially the things and people you may tend to take for granted. Let your loved ones know how much you appreciate them and how special they are to you.

Do everything in your power to enhance the lives of others, and help them attain bliss and harmony in their own lives. Seek the truth and divine value in all things and in all people.

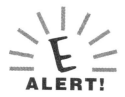

ALERT!

You cannot truly pursue spiritual peace and contentment if old wounds from negative personal experiences continue to plague you. It is important to heal old emotional and psychological wounds. If possible, repair damaged relationships. Otherwise, move on. Either way, do not carry around grudges or negative feelings. Forgive those who have wronged you, in order to encourage their healing as well as yours.

Encourage your own spiritual wellness and healing, and that of others. Seek ways to heal old emotional wounds, and recover from past traumas. Therapy may be useful, or perhaps a support group—even if it is just an informal support group consisting of friends and loved ones.

Treat People Right

Tantrics of ancient times believed that it was of utmost importance to live an honorable and respectful life. This meant always acting in a moral and ethical manner and treating others with love, respect, and kindness. This continues to be a major cornerstone of Tantric principles today.

Everyone Is an Important Life Force

Later in this book you will learn about the importance of treating your partner as a god or goddess. And while your partner should hold a special place in your life, it is equally important to treat everyone else—from family members to total strangers—with a certain level of respect, in a way befitting a Tantric. For example Tantrics believe:

- All creatures embody an important life force that is to be respected and treasured.
- You should speak honestly and respectfully to others, and truly listen to them and hear what they are trying to say.
- You should approach everyone with acceptance, awareness, and respect for their important place in life and the world.

Live a Moral Life

In many Tantric communities, it is considered very important for all people to conduct themselves in a moral and civilized manner, one that encourages peace and bliss in the world. You should act in a way that is not disruptive to the world, but encourages harmony and peace.

As a Tantric, you should always behave in a way befitting a god or goddess and never bring negative energy to yourself or those around you. Always have respect for yourself, your spirit, and your body. Treat loved ones with unconditional love, respect, and loyalty.

Embrace a New Outlook on Life

In accordance with your new Tantric approach, you will find that you take a new outlook on life. Welcome this fresh perspective on the universe! It is a rare gift. Few people get the valuable opportunity to feel as if they have been given the ability to totally reinvent their outlook on life, to be "reborn." Do not let this chance at a new beginning go to waste.

Relax your boundaries and explore new things—uncharted territories in your relationships and unexplored parts of the world around you. Resist feelings of guilt, fear, embarrassment, or other negative factors that have weighed you down and prevented you from experiencing life to its fullest. Abandon old notions that taint your view of sacred acts such as sexual unions. Recognize that this beautiful act is a natural and spiritual event, one that is positive and joyful, not bad or dirty.

Expand your visions and goals for yourself, your loved ones, your community, and the world. Encourage your own dreams and those of others.

Realize that you are one with the Earth, the heavens, and the universe. Welcome and embrace this oneness. Do everything in your power to enable a harmonious union and to avoid disrupting the harmony of this existence.

Accept Your Newfound Openness

As you progress in your Tantric journey, you will find yourself becoming more open to the world and the people around you. You will be receptive to new experiences, relationships, and feelings. This is a good thing, as it allows you to expand your life's journey and broaden your horizons, allowing you to enjoy many exciting and pleasurable things.

However, being open and receptive to new things can be scary and foreign, especially if you have always been cautious and tended to take the "safe" road before.

Realize that new does not equal bad. It is natural and good to try new things and welcome new experiences. Even if you do not ultimately decide to make all of these new experiences a regular part of your life, you have enriched your existence just by branching out into new areas.

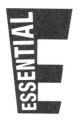

Some ancient Tantrics believed that in order to have a completely full and satisfying life, one must explore every possible activity, including (or perhaps especially) those viewed as sinful by the general population. So some ancient Tantrics actually sought out the most scandalous activities possible. That's an extreme, but being just a bit "naughty" occasionally can be refreshing.

If you had previously become accustomed to stifling your feelings or denying your natural urges, this new freedom to express yourself and embrace life's wonders can be disconcerting and maybe even frightening. You may have the urge to put up your guard, or to build emotional walls to keep you from feeling so vulnerable. Resist this instinct. Vulnerability is a good thing in this case. It allows you to communicate freely with loved ones and experience stronger connections than ever before. And with your partner, this openness will help you express your needs and desires, and be totally honest in your thoughts, words, and actions. Your partner will be pleasantly surprised by this transformation and will appreciate you trusting her with your most treasured secrets. This most likely will motivate your partner, in turn, to be more open with you and make him feel free to express himself in a more significant way.

Granting yourself permission to be completely open and receptive to Tantra and to your partner will fill you with a powerful sense of freedom and peace. You will no longer need to worry about shame, hesitation, embarrassment, or any of those other things that may be holding you back. This will open many exciting new days for you and pave the way for countless new experiences and fantastic journeys.

Share Tantric Teachings with Others

More than likely, Tantra will bring so much happiness and positive energy into your life that you will want to sing its praises from the rooftops. At the very least, you will want to rave about it to everyone you know. This is only natural, and it is an admirable thing.

Proceed with Caution

However, you should keep in mind that not everyone is as interested in Tantra as you are. While some people may be receptive to hearing your insights, others will quickly become bored or disinterested or may even cut you off or turn away. Do not take this personally and don't let it discourage you. Nor should this cloud your view of this person. The time must be right for an individual to be fully receptive to considering new ways of thinking. Perhaps this is not a good time in this person's life, and he is not in a place where he is ready to embrace change of any kind. Or perhaps his view may be clouded by preconceived notions he has of Tantra based on misinformation and misconceptions.

For those who are receptive to hearing about Tantra, approach the situation with careful thought. Remember that different people learn in different ways. Some may want to hear about every tiny detail, possibly including the rich history of Tantra and all of the important (and often colorful) gurus and other notable figures involved in the evolution of Tantra. Others want the short-and-sweet version: how Tantra works, where they can learn it, and how it can change their lives.

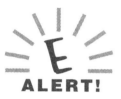

ALERT!

Keep in mind, too, that although your newly recharged sexual relationship is a wonderful thing, not everyone wants to hear about your steamy sex life. Your grandmother, for example, could probably do without your bedroom recaps. In some cases, you may want to tread lightly when describing these particular benefits of Tantra.

Spread the Message Effectively

If someone is truly eager to hear about your experiences with Tantra, be open and honest with her. Tell her about all of the good things Tantra has brought to your life—and also be frank about any challenges or problems you may have faced along the way to spiritual enlightenment. Encourage her to go through the same process that you yourself went through, in evaluating your needs and determining what type of Tantra was right for you.

If your friend is more of a practical, logical person, you may need to introduce abstract spiritual concepts slowly, so as not to overwhelm him or scare him off. Illustrate the tangible, practical benefits you have gotten from Tantra. On the other hand, if your friend tends toward the more spiritual and is into cosmic awareness, you can be a bit looser with the "New Age" stuff.

And if the person is someone who is very comfortable with her sexuality and has no problem with frank talks about sex, you may (if you feel comfortable) share with her some of the ways that Tantra has enhanced your sexual relations and strengthened your intimate connection with your partner. (If your friend is a guy, especially a young guy, often just the mention of a hotter sex life can often grab his attention and make him eager to hear more.)

Whatever your approach, you should not come on too strong or appear too aggressive to promote Tantra. This will tend to scare people off and make them even less receptive to hearing about the subject in the future. It is understandable—and admirable—that you want to let everyone in on "your little secret," but if you come across too strongly, people may view you as a fanatic—or even worse, fear you are trying to "recruit" them, as with some kind of cult.

Be a Supportive Tantra Coach

Once your friend has taken the first steps and is firm in his desire to learn, you can be helpful by offering advice as to the best way for him to explore the Tantric teachings. Knowing your friend's personality and preferences, you will probably be able to suggest a few strategies or resources that might best complement his learning style.

You can offer to accompany your friend to a Tantra workshop, if you both feel comfortable with that. This may be especially helpful if both of you are single (and of opposite genders) and your friend is reluctant to attend a workshop alone for fear of being paired up with a stranger. Prior to the event, think back to your fears or concerns before attending your first Tantra event. Most likely, your friend has the same thoughts, so do your best to address her concerns and reassure her about the experience.

You can of course also share any resources you have gathered in your quest for Tantric knowledge, such as books, CDs, or other materials you have found especially helpful. If you liked these particular materials and found them helpful, it is likely that your friend will too.

Another way to be a supportive "Tantra coach" is to make some of your Tantra rituals a fun activity you and your friend can do together. Perhaps you can do your yoga and breathing routines together, or help each other decorate your individual sacred spaces.

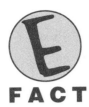

FACT

Female friends often enjoy going on "Tantra shopping sprees" together, helping to stock up on aromatic candles, romantic outfits, and maybe a few little bedroom accessories. Make this into a fun girls' day out.

What is the best way you can be a great Tantra coach? By setting a good example. If you feel happy and fulfilled on the inside, it will surely show on the outside. It will probably be obvious that Tantra has transformed you into a content, blissful, balanced (and yes, sexually satisfied) person. As a result, you will barely need to say a word to promote the wonders of Tantra. Your demeanor will speak for itself, and people will be eager to hear your secret for attaining such an enviable state.

Chapter 15

Monogamy and Safe Sex

When it comes to sex, the word *safe* isn't exactly a turn-on. People tend to like things wild and risqué in the bedroom. Safety is often seen as synonymous with "boring." However, the days of "free love" with no regrets have passed. Like it or not, safety is an important consideration these days when it comes to sex. However, safe does not necessarily need to equal boring. With a little planning and some precautions, you can have a wild and exciting sex life while still keeping yourself safe.

Monogamy Basics

These days, in light of the rising AIDS infection rate and other sexually transmitted diseases, most people have at least a basic knowledge about monogamy and safe sex. But, just to make sure, it is probably a good idea to do a quick overview of the basics. Monogamy refers to the practice of having sex with only one partner. You do not need to be married to be monogamous. Many single people are in committed monogamous relationships.

Reasons for Monogamy

There are many different reasons why people practice a monogamous lifestyle. For many people, this is just what seems like the natural thing to do. For women especially, it is often an automatic thing—they simply take it for granted that they and their partner will be faithful to each other. (Of course, if both partners are not on the same page when it comes to this issue, there can be major problems. So good communication is the key to successful monogamy.)

People also practice monogamy for moral or religious reasons. Some people, especially women, believe they will be viewed as having loose morals if they have sex with several different partners.

Other people practice monogamy because it is just comfortable and convenient. They like the stability and familiarity of being with the same partner continuously. As many women point out, it can often take a while to feel comfortable disrobing in front of a new partner, so the idea of working up the courage to get naked for the first time in front of a long series of partners is not very appealing.

Monogamy in History

It can be tough to trace the roots of monogamy throughout history, mainly because the meaning of the word has changed over the years. Initially, *monogamy* was a term that simply meant the practice of taking only one spouse (generally a wife) at a time. As a result, many married men who technically practiced monogamy because they only had one wife were also carrying on numerous relationships with their mistresses at the same time.

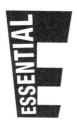

There are many people who believe you can practice safe sex while still enjoying many partners if you are not in a committed monogamous relationship. The hot new catchphrase for this approach is "responsible nonmonogamy," although medical experts are quick to point out that any sexual activity involving multiple partners involves at least some inherent risks.

Today, the term is used more broadly to refer to a couple in a committed relationship (which does not necessarily involve marriage) who only have sex with each other.

Throughout history, different cultures and religions have taken vastly different views on monogamy. For Catholics, of course, the final word on monogamy is literally written in stone, in the form of the commandment dictating "Thou shalt not commit adultery." Interestingly enough, though, even within the Catholic texts there are contradictions: The Bible contains many references to men who have numerous extramarital consorts.

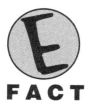

FACT

In many cultures, the top priority for a man—especially for members of royalty—was having a male heir. Men commonly had sex with numerous women in pursuing that goal, especially if the wife did not give birth to a son. In these cases, infidelity was a nonissue, as it was considered far less important than the man's quest for a male heir.

A common approach to sex throughout history in many cultures has been that the man would have a single wife, with some discreet affairs on the side. Monogamy was not a huge issue in many societies, except in certain strict religious faiths where it was specifically prohibited.

Couple as Guru

An important tenet when it comes to Tantric sexuality (specifically under Neo-Tantra beliefs) is the idea that romantic partners serve as each other's guru. Therefore, the partners need to have total and complete trust and faith in each other. It is critical in a Tantric relationship to have unwavering faith in your partner, to believe that he or she has your well-being and spiritual happiness utmost in his or her mind.

If it is established (or assumed) in the relationship that both partners will remain faithful and one partner violates that rule, this can result in a major breach of trust. The partner who has been cheated on may feel betrayed, and feel that his or her partner has violated the sacred trust of the relationship. In essence, the actual infidelity is secondary to the more important issue of trust and honesty.

Truth and Vulnerability

A core issue when discussing the topic of fidelity and monogamy is trust. For many people, it can be difficult to fully trust someone else. This is especially true in cases where the person has previously been hurt or betrayed by a lover or someone else he or she trusted. So it can take a lot of time, patience, and effort to establish a trusting relationship.

As far as sex goes, while casual sex can be no sweat, it generally takes a lot more work to establish a committed sexual relationship based on a foundation of trust. This requires both parties to break down the walls they may have put up around their emotional core. They must allow themselves to be open and vulnerable, which can be scary—if not downright terrifying—for many people.

With a committed sexual relationship, there are two issues in play. First, you are opening yourself up to your partner emotionally and trusting that person to protect your emotional well-being. But you are also opening yourself up sexually, perhaps revealing your most secret sexual thoughts and desires. You might eventually feel comfortable enough to reveal thoughts or fantasies you have not shared with many other people—or perhaps have never shared with anyone before now. You may also work up the nerve to engage in sexual activities you were afraid to try before. This can leave you feeling exposed and vulnerable, and force you to rely on the trust you have in your partner to guard those secrets.

For many people, this is the basis behind the desire for monogamy. Reaching this point of trust and vulnerability with another person is a huge accomplishment, one that does not come easily. When you have achieved this state, you share a powerful intimate bond, one that can be tough or impossible to replicate with another person.

If this is your view of your relationship, it can be devastating to imagine that your partner has disregarded this safe and trusting state that you worked so hard to achieve. To you, it is not just the point of a physical betrayal—your partner has also crushed your trust and possibly destroyed the foundation of the relationship. Your partner has made you regret allowing yourself to become open and vulnerable, which can be a huge setback to overcome.

Of course, there is the added issue of your partner's disregard for your physical well-being, if he or she had sex with another person and did not take proper precautions, thereby leaving you at risk for various sexually transmitted diseases.

Safe Sex

There are many precautions you can take to make your sex life safer. These days, most sexually active adults are familiar with most of the basic safe sex techniques. (Most public schools have introduced this topic as part of their health curriculum, so even most teenagers today have been taught the basics about sex-related health risks.)

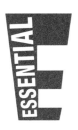

Although it is common for people today to use the phrase "safe sex," this term is actually frowned upon by many health professionals and sex educators. This is because it implies that you can make sex completely safe—and, of course, it is generally accepted that no sexual activity (except masturbation) can ever be 100 percent safe. Therefore, experts tend to prefer the term "*safer* sex."

The Safest Techniques

Of course, as medical experts are quick to point out, the only guaranteed way to be totally safe is through abstinence (although masturbation presumably also falls under the totally safe category). Short of abstinence, mutual masturbation and sensual massage are probably the next best things, from a safety standpoint, as there are no bodily fluids exchanged.

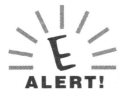

ALERT!

When using condoms, be very careful about any lubricants or gels you use at the same time. Certain types of gels—mainly oil-based ones—can damage the latex, causing the condom to break. Look for water-based gels specifically designed for use in conjunction with condoms.

Condoms are probably the most popular method of sexual protection (of course, they also provide the added benefit of preventing unwanted pregnancy). In the past, condoms often got a bad rap because men complained that they were constricting and reduced sexual sensations. However, condoms have come a long way in recent years—today, there are lots of exciting types, including ribbed varieties, condoms designed especially for the female partner's pleasure—even condoms that are flavored or glow in the dark. For the sake of convenience, many major condom manufacturers offer a variety pack, which allows you to try several different types of condoms and decide which one(s) you like best. Talk about a fun "market research" assignment!

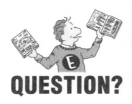

QUESTION?

What type of condom offers the best protection?
Lubricated latex condoms are generally considered the best and most effective at protecting against sexually transmitted diseases. Lambskin varieties can be riskier, as they are not viewed to be as effective in preventing the transmission of disease.

Be sure to use condoms for oral sex, too, not just for intercourse. Bodily fluids can be transmitted by oral/genital contact, which can lead to the spread of HIV and other sexually transmitted diseases.

The most common problem with condoms is that they are used incorrectly. They can be unexpectedly tricky to put on, especially in the heat of passion, so it is a good idea to practice a few times beforehand, especially if you are inexperienced with condoms. Be sure to put it on right-side out, and leave sufficient extra space at the tip to allow for ejaculation without breakage (many condoms have a built-in reservoir for this purpose).

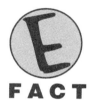

FACT

You should also use condoms on any dildos or similar sex toys you might be using. In addition to helping prevent the spread of disease, this will also make it easier to keep these items clean and protect them from damage.

Least Effective Techniques

One of the least effective safe sex techniques? The withdrawal method—or "pulling out"—which is especially popular with teenagers who mistakenly believe they can use it to avoid unwanted pregnancy. This technique involves the man removing his penis from the woman right before he feels like he is going to ejaculate. The problem with this plan is obvious—many men have trouble gauging exactly when they are going to ejaculate, and even if they do recognize the warning signs, they are often unable or unwilling to put on the brakes and pull out in time. Even if they are successful in pulling out before climax, that is often still too late because some seminal fluid is excreted even before the point of actual ejaculation.

Douching is another strategy popular with teenagers (and sexual novices) in a misguided effort to prevent the spread of disease and unwanted pregnancy. Unfortunately, this technique is a dismal failure on both counts. Douching immediately after sex can actually push the sperm and seminal fluid further up the vaginal canal faster than would normally happen, which as a result can actually *increase* the risk or pregnancy or disease transmission. In theory, then, this would be a practice for people trying to get pregnant—although most doctors would not actually recommend it, since this can also make it more likely that harmful bacteria and other material would be pushed into the vaginal canal.

Safe Can Be Fun

In most areas of life, *safe* and *fun* are words that mean exact opposites to most people. But when it comes to sex, safety does not have to be boring. In fact, thanks to modern sexual aids, it is possible to make safe sex more fun than ever. There are endless varieties of "fun" condoms—including those designed to enhance the woman's pleasure—that can allow you to enjoy hot sex while still taking the important precautions.

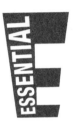

To make safe sex exciting, create a safe sex "treasure chest" that you keep handy near your bed or sensual space. Stock up on fun sexual aids like condoms in fun colors and flavors, lubricated gels, and more. Make it a fun game to let your partner choose his assortments of "safe sex surprises" before you get down to business.

Making Monogamy Exciting

The biggest challenge when it comes to monogamy is keeping things exciting—maintaining that air of mystery or sense of newness you experience with a new partner is essential. For many people, the risk of infidelity starts to increase when one or both partners begins to feel like they are in a rut, when they get bored with doing the same old thing with the same person over and over again.

The good news is, it is easy to get yourself out of that rut and make things exciting again without seeking other partners. You have taken a big first step by learning about Tantric sex, which will help spice things up in the bedroom. But you can also take other simple steps, like having sex in new positions or a new environment. To capture the excitement of having sex with someone new (while having sex with your existing partner) try role-playing or dressing up in wild costumes. As long as you are both okay with it, it is fine to pretend to be other people—although it's usually advisable to pick an imaginary person, or an unattainable one like a famous celebrity or rock star, as opposed to someone you know. Incorporating a friend or acquaintance into your fantasies can make your partner worry that you harbor secret desires for that person. Be very careful about this, even if your partner assures you he or she can handle it. Many people are not quite as secure as they may think. Admitting that you harbor a secret attraction for, say, your dentist is something your partner is not likely to take lightly—and may provoke feelings of jealousy or insecurity. Bottom line: Tread very lightly. Unless you are 100 percent sure your partner can handle it, keep any secret crushes on friends or acquaintances to yourself.

Monogamy Versus Polyamory

A popular misconception about Tantric sex is the notion that it involves people having wild and reckless group sex at orgies and other sexual free-for-all events. While it is true that many Tantric practitioners do engage in wild sexual activities, this is an individual choice. Many Tantrics are focused on enhancing and strengthening that treasured romantic bond with one special partner. For most people, the main goal of studying Tantra, from a sexual standpoint, is to establish and nurture that intimate connection with one specific partner—to strengthen your bond as a couple. It is in keeping with the whole "union of forces" idea, the yin and yang concept upon which Tantra is based.

Polyamory

There is a relatively small segment of the Tantric community that practices a lifestyle known as *polyamory*—meaning, engaging in sexual relations with multiple partners.

People in a polyamorous lifestyle often have the viewpoint that people were destined to engage in a sexually open and flexible lifestyle. They often believe that monogamy is actually the more unnatural lifestyle choice and that, even if it is admirable in theory, it is nearly always impossible to maintain (perhaps evidenced by the high rates of infidelity among married couples).

It is tough to pinpoint a "typical" polyamorous couple, since (like any other couple) these couples tend to make up their own rules and circumstances according to their own needs and desires. It is important, however, to distinguish between polyamory and the basic "swinging" lifestyle. There is a difference. Polyamory in Tantra is about more than having multiple sex partners—there's a spiritual and love (not necessarily romantic love) connection that isn't a focal point in garden-variety multiple-partner sex. People who practice a polyamorous lifestyle will generally become offended if you refer to them as "swingers."

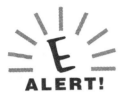

ALERT!

Do not confuse polyamory with polygamy. Polyamory means having sexual relations with partners outside of your relationship (with your partner's knowledge). Polygamy, on the other hand, is the practice of being married to more than one person at the same time.

Polyamory's Roots

Polyamory dates back to ancient origins, when it was common for men—especially those in the upper echelons of society—to have sex with many women, sometimes in rapid succession or at the same time. Often, the man would have a group of consorts that he would rank according to their background, physical attributes, or other criteria. He would then make love to them in succession, starting with the lowest-ranking, allowing the highest-ranking consort to have the esteemed final position. (Customarily, despite having all of this sex with many women in a row, the man may not have ejaculated a single time, in keeping with the tradition of not wasting his valuable energy fluids.)

Types of Polyamorous Relationships

It is important to distinguish between polyamorous relationships and affairs. While it is true that married people having sex with someone other than their spouse does technically meet the definition of infidelity, those who practice the polyamorous lifestyle are quick to point out the differences. In this situation, there is no "cheating" because no deception is involved. One of the primary ground rules in these situations is that everything is done upfront and with full disclosure. There are several different varieties of polyamorous situations:

- In a common approach, couples engage in threesomes with a partner they both choose and approve of. They may keep this same partner for ongoing repeated encounters, or choose a new partner for each encounter.
- Taking the threesome a step further, they may engage in a foursome with another couple, where all parties are actively participating in the encounter.
- It is also possible that the partners will each separately engage in sex with other people, while their partner does not participate (but may observe).
- In some cases, the couple may actually establish a type of group relationship, almost like a communal partnership, where they take turns engaging in sex with partners within their tight-knit group, but do not welcome outsiders as partners.
- Some polyamorous couples in the Tantric community regularly host and/or attend retreats or get-togethers specifically designed for "the sharing of love." At these events, partners may select other people to have sex with, possibly while their partner joins in or watches.

Chapter 16

Toys, Props, and Extras

Even the most sexually satisfied and adventurous couples can benefit from experimenting with some bedroom props and accessories. Although many people are initially hesitant to first experiment with sex toys, in the end they are almost always glad they took this step. Toys and props can add a new level of thrill to your sex life, and many couples find themselves becoming big fans of these adult toys.

Toys and Their Role in Tantra

Some people incorrectly assume that sex toys may be discouraged or looked down upon by Tantra teachers and gurus. In fact, it is just the opposite. Tantra welcomes anything that helps a couple enrich their sex life and strengthen their intimate bond. The only caveat would be that the couple needs to make sure they do not become too focused on the toys and props, to the point where these things distract from the couple's sensual and spiritual connection, rather than enhancing it.

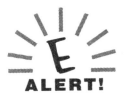

ALERT!

If one partner is strongly opposed to the use of sex toys in the bedroom and the other person exerts pressure on her or ignores her feelings, this may actually end up hurting the relationship. It is better to be patient and wait until your partner is ready to take this step.

Introducing Toys to the Bedroom

Ideally, both partners are equally interested in using toys or introducing them to the couple's sexual repertoire. If you both have an existing interest in toys and props, you have a huge head start in this area. Unfortunately, it is somewhat rare that both partners are so perfectly in sync when it comes to this issue. More likely, one partner has been contemplating the use of toys and props, and has been trying to figure out a way to broach the subject with their partner.

This should be done carefully and with some planning beforehand. You will want to have your "sales pitch" thought out in detail beforehand, so you can make your best and most convincing case in favor of props. This is one of those situations where it is all in the presentation. Depending on how you present the idea and explain your reason for wanting to take this new step, you can make or break the whole thing.

Reluctance by the Female

Often, women may be afraid or uncomfortable with the idea of experimenting with sex toys. There are several reasons for this. A primary factor is that many women were given negative ideas and attitudes about sex as young girls. They may have gotten the idea that even intercourse itself was bad or dirty—so, obviously, adding a foreign object to the equation really ups the "bad" factor.

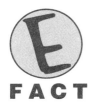

FACT

Sex toys—especially vibrators designed for clitoral stimulation—can provide a valuable service to a woman's sex life. For women who have difficulty achieving orgasm, a sex toy can help by allowing her to explore various movements and sensations until she finds the ones that are most pleasing to her. Soon she may become very familiar with her specific "route to orgasm."

Ideally, your partner has some female friends who are open to having some frank sexual discussions with her. If they discuss their own experiences with sex toys, it will help your partner realize that this is not something dirty or evil, and that lots of "normal" women enjoy using sex toys.

If you can't enlist the help of her chatty female friends, try scouring some women's magazines for articles mentioning sex toys. Again, this will help her realize that many other women regularly use and enjoy sex toys.

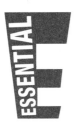

When you are first attempting to convince your female partner to try sex toys, it can be a bad idea to show her X-rated pictures or movies depicting women using these toys. This can easily backfire on you, as it may reinforce her beliefs that only "bad" women—promiscuous women and porn stars—use these types of toys.

Women who are shy or sexually self-conscious may also be timid about trying sex toys. Tip: if a woman is reluctant to masturbate while you watch, it is a likely bet that she will also be hesitant about using a sex toy in front of you. The key here is to take things slow; don't put too much pressure on her. If you act too eager about watching her with this toy, she may feel like she needs to put on a show for you, which can be intimidating. To avoid this, it can be helpful for you to allow her to practice using the toy in privacy by herself a few times, so she becomes more comfortable before using it with you watching her.

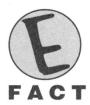

FACT

A worldwide study conducted by Durex in 2004 found that 27 percent of respondents owned a vibrator or intimate massager. That figure rises to more than a third of both twenty-five to thirty-four year olds and those in the forty-five-plus age group.

Women may also be reluctant to try sex toys simply because they are unfamiliar and scary. Although she may be embarrassed to admit this, your partner may be afraid that a sex toy may be painful, or that she won't know how to use it correctly. In this case, it can be helpful to look for toys that are packaged with manuals or illustrated guides explaining how to use the product. Again, you should allow her to review this material (and, if she wishes, to practice using the toy) alone if she feels more comfortable that way.

If your female partner is slightly reluctant or nervous about using sex toys for the first time, but still summons up the guts to make her "debut" in front of you, do not do anything that would make her regret it. Proceed very slowly and cautiously and follow her lead. If you rush things or appear overeager, you will simply increase her anxiety and possibly cause her to change her mind completely. The good news? If you control your enthusiasm and have a little patience, it is very likely that your partner will quickly discover the joys of these products and will soon be using them (with or without you) with gusto.

Reluctance by the Male

Men are often more willing to try new things in the bedroom than women, but this may not be true when it comes to sex toys—specifically vibrators and dildos. Some men may feel insulted that their partner needs what the man might view as a "replacement penis." This may make them feel insecure, worried that their woman is not happy with their performance. They may also feel insulted by what they perceive as a criticism of their manhood.

If this is the case, it is important for the woman to provide reassurance that she is very satisfied with her man and that she loves everything he does to please her. It is important for her to stress that the sex toy is not to replace the man or to compensate for any kind of shortcomings on his part, but rather to enhance the good sexual foundation they have already established.

Obviously, if the man has any type of insecurities about his performance, it is critical for the woman to avoid appearing overly excited by the sex toy. She does not want to seem so obsessed with it that her partner feels overlooked or unneeded. Should her male partner display any sign of insecurity during a sexual encounter, the woman should immediately abandon the sex toy and direct her full focus to the man, reassuring him that he is her priority.

Types of Sex Toys

To people new to the world of sex toys, it can be shocking—and maybe a bit overwhelming—to discover just how many different types of sex toys are out there. It seems like there are new toys and sex aids hitting the market every day, from balls and beads to creams and "cock rings." While it would take too long to discuss every type of sex toy, here is a primer on the most common kinds of adult toys.

Vibrators

The vibrator is probably the most common and most well known type of sex toy. A vibrator is especially designed to stimulate a specific part of the female anatomy—mainly, the clitoris. This is important, since many women achieve orgasm primarily through clitoral stimulation—and for some women, clitoral stimulation is a must in order to climax. Unlike dildos, vibrators generally do not have that penislike appearance. In fact, many vibrators are small and flexible (at least at the tip) in order to allow for easier access to the clitoris and greater flexibility of movement.

There is no one "typical" type of vibrator, though, because they are available in countless shapes and sizes.

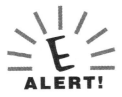

Contrary to popular misconception, vibrators are not intended to be inserted or used inside the body. In fact, because of the unusual design of some vibrators, they can feel awkward or even painful when inserted vaginally. If you want a toy that does double-duty (vibrating and insertable) look for a vibrating dildo.

There are several things to consider when choosing a vibrator:

- **Noise:** The stereotypical vibrator is very noisy, so it can be challenging to use discreetly, especially if you live with roommates or parents. Many newer models are specifically designed to be very quiet.
- **Size:** Vibrators are available in a wide array of sizes, from pocket-sized to jumbo units. The smaller ones are easier to carry discreetly, while the larger models generally offer more features.
- **Price:** Just because you are on a tight budget doesn't mean you must forgo vibrators. You can find the smaller basic models for under $20. On the other hand, if price is no object, you can splurge on a fancy high-tech model that costs $150 or more.
- **Speed:** Ideally, your vibrator offers a selection of varying speeds. It is generally a good idea to start off with the slowest speed, especially if you are inexperienced with a vibrator, so that the experience isn't overwhelming. Most women then gradually "step up" to higher speeds as they become more comfortable and more aroused.

- **Extra features:** Many vibrators, especially the more expensive models, offer extra features. These may include the ability to be used in the water, multiple "heads" that can stimulate several different areas (as in, the clitoris and G-spot) at the same time, or an attached butt plug.

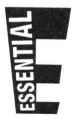

If you will be traveling with your vibrator, be sure to remove the batteries beforehand so that it does not cause an embarrassing scene by turning on accidentally. When traveling by plane, you should pack your vibrator and other toys in your checked luggage, for added privacy.

Dildos

Dildos are penislike toys designed to be inserted vaginally (and possibly anally). The traditional dildo was pretty cut-and-dry: an implement that resembled a penis in general size, shape, and appearance that was meant to be inserted into the vagina or anus to provide roughly the same sensation as penetration by a penis.

But today the dildo has come a long way from its basic roots. Modern versions have all kind of enhancements like ridges, bumps, or even veins and other features designed to make it more closely resemble an actual penis. There are "double-ended dildos" designed for use by two people at the same time. There are also vibrating dildos, designed to do the work of a dildo and a vibrator in one convenient toy.

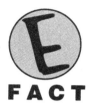

FACT

When using a dildo or similar toy, it can be helpful to soak it in warm water or oil for a while beforehand. This helps soften up the toy, and it also makes it warm enough to prevent any uncomfortable cold shocks.

Enhancing Creams

A new type of sexual aid that has been gaining popularity lately is "enhancing creams." These products come in gel or cream form and are designed to be rubbed directly on the genitals for added stimulation. They usually provide a quick (and often short-lived) tingling sensation in the area on which they are applied. The effectiveness of these products varies by brand and ingredients.

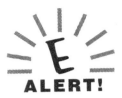

ALERT!

When trying an enhancing cream for the first time, be sure to start with a tiny amount until you gauge its effects. Using a low-quality cream (or an excessive amount of any cream) can often cause a burning sensation that many people find uncomfortable or even painful. It goes without saying that you do not want to risk experiencing these sensations in sensitive areas.

Just for Men

While vibrators and other women-specific products may be the first things to spring to mind when envisioning sex toys, there is a whole category of toys designed especially with men in mind. Here are a few of the most common male sex toys:

- **Rings:** Generally known as penis rings (or the more X-rated term of "cock rings"), these are usually made of a rubbery-type material able to stretch over just about any size penis. They are designed to provide constriction, which helps a man maintain an erection. The fancier models are adorned with extras like beads and bumps, which can help enhance the female partner's pleasure during intercourse. Penis rings are also available in a vibrating variety. Note: Penis rings should not be worn for too long (say more than a half hour) because constricting the penis for an extended period of time can cause negative effects.

- **Pumps:** These are another type of product designed to help men maintain an erection for longer periods of time. The pump usually features a "sleeve" made from a rubbery jellylike material, which is placed over the penis. Using the accompanying pump, the man can get a sensation similar to that he would get from a vigorous session of oral or manual stimulation.
- **Oral simulators:** These are products that are placed over the penis and designed to mimic the sucking sensation of oral sex.
- **Fake vaginas:** A product growing in popularity is the fake vagina. Some of the higher-priced models can have a very lifelike feel, and the bestselling varieties are often modeled after the actual genitals of porn stars. These can come in handy when the man desires intercourse but his female partner is not available or not in the mood. Obviously, the man should make sure his partner has no objection to his using this "vaginal stand-in" for his sexual satisfaction.

Anal Toys

There is a whole section of adult toys designed specifically for anal use. The most common anal toys are known as "butt plugs." These are soft, flexible implements, usually made of a rubbery jellylike material, which are somewhat similar to dildos but with a slightly different shape. Available in a variety of sizes—including small versions designed especially for "beginners"—these can be a good way to gradually work your way up to actual anal sex involving penile penetration. Some butt plugs are also designed to fit into specially designed harnesses that can be worn by the woman in order to anally penetrate her male partner.

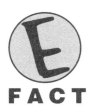

FACT

When using any type of anal toy, it is important to take the same precautions you would for anal sex in general. Mainly, be sure to use lots of lubrication for comfort and easier insertion. Also, never insert anything into the vagina or other areas immediately after it has been in the anal area without cleaning it first.

Another popular type of anal toy is anal beads. Anal beads are nothing new—they have been used in Oriental sex practices for thousands of years. (They differ from Ben Wa balls, which are much larger and are inserted into the vagina.) Anal beads can be used by men or women, alone or with their partner. The general concept is similar to a string of pearls, although anal beads are available in a wide variety of sizes and textures. They are inserted, one at a time, into the anus and then pulled out at a desired moment—usually near the point of orgasm, or simultaneously with the climax.

Props

Aside from actual sex toys, there are many other items you can use to spice up your sex life. Some of the most common sex props include dusters or anything with feathers that can provide a tickling sensation. More adventurous couples often use more risqué props like handcuffs, straps, or other bondage-type items. Swings and harnesses can also be exciting props, although they can prove challenging at first.

You may also choose props that complement your particular sexual fantasy. For example, couples who like to enact a principal/schoolgirl fantasy scenario may use props like a desk and textbooks. And you thought a chemistry book couldn't be sexy!

With a little creativity and imagination, you can devise ways to use "mainstream" items (as in, things not designed with sex in mind) as props to incorporate into your sex life. The benefit of this is that you can buy these items at many locations, not just sex shops, and you won't be embarrassed to have friends or relatives spot these innocent-looking items in your home.

Clothing

Clothing is a very popular type of sexual enhancer. Obviously, there is the bedroom staple: sexy lingerie. And with the popularity of stores like Victoria's Secret in malls across the country, hot lingerie is available to women everywhere. But some couples prefer sensual clothing that is not quite so overtly sexual—things like silk robes, velvet pajamas, etc.

Couples can also enjoy clothing that fits with their particular fantasies or turn-ons: a French maid outfit, schoolgirl uniform, nurse uniform, etc.

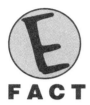

FACT

If you are going through the trouble of dressing up in special clothing for your romantic encounter, be sure you have enough time to enjoy seeing each other wearing it (and, more importantly, slowly removing it). Clothing and other props aren't really intended for two-minute quickies, so save them for when you can enjoy a longer encounter.

Food and Wine

Sex toys and props are not limited to things you can wear or insert in various parts of your body. It can also involve things you eat and drink. For many people, food and wine play a pivotal role in the whole romantic experience.

Aphrodisiacs

We all know that eating certain foods can be a sensual experience. Picture a luscious, decadent assortment of rich chocolates. And there are the stereotypical aphrodisiacs like oysters and the above-mentioned chocolates. But "fantasy foods" can vary from one couple to another. For people with a sweet tooth, candies and cake can help set the mood. On the other hand, fitness buffs may find that a health smoothie really gets their sexual juices flowing. Tradition may also play a role: Couples often get turned on by foods that hold special significance in their relationship—something that reminds them of the meal they shared on their first date, for example.

Alcohol

We all know the stereotypical romantic scene, straight out of the movies, that features a bottled of pricey champagne chilling in a bucket on ice. And it is true that champagne—or whatever type of alcohol you prefer—can help set a romantic mood. Many people like to enjoy a glass or two of wine to help them relax. For the sexually shy or skittish, a small amount of alcohol can be helpful in loosening the inhibitions. Plus, it can be romantic to share a glass of champagne—and perhaps make a toast to a happy future together.

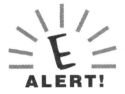

ALERT!

When it comes to alcohol and romantic encounters, watch out for a few pitfalls. Engaging in sex while severely drunk is never a good idea. And if you realize that you or your partner can *only* enjoy sex after drinking, that's a red flag. And obviously you should never have sex if your partner is so inebriated as to not be aware of his or her actions.

Setting the Scene

Often, when it comes to food and romance, it is not so much a matter of *what* you eat as *how* you eat it. It can be sexy to take turns feeding each other—try a romantic staple like strawberries dipped in whipped cream, or take turns experimenting with your own selections.

If using a table, appearance counts. Adorn the table with a lace or silk tablecloth, if possible, and break out your best dinnerware. Nothing kills a romantic mood faster than paper plates and plastic cups.

Or use your partner's body as a buffet table. Have her lie flat on her back and then place various foods (obviously nothing too hot or cold) on specific parts of her body.

Food as Sex Toy

Of course, you can also work the food into your sex life in a more active, direct way. Some couples like to use food items as an actual sex toy by placing them in or on the erogenous zones. A common example: eating whipped cream off your partner's private parts. Or using a cucumber or similar food as a makeshift dildo (only after thoroughly washing it, of course). It can also be exciting to use an ice cube in your sexual routine. Putting something warm or cold in your mouth before performing oral sex on your partner can create some unique sensations. Be creative: Some women have tried placing a glazed donut around their man's penis and eating it off as part of oral sex.

Buying Sex Toys

Even people who have no qualms about using sex toys may be a bit uncomfortable actually buying them. Thankfully, the days when you needed to venture into a seedy sex shop to buy your adult toys are long gone. Today, you can buy adult toys and props in complete privacy from the comfort of your own home, via mail order and the thousands of online retailers. The major adult retailers take their customers' privacy very seriously and will take great care to ship products discreetly.

You can find leads of some reputable adult toy retailers and online stores in the Resources section of this book.

Chapter 17

Books and Videos

When it comes to sex in general—and Tantric sex specifically—it seems like you can never study too hard. (On the plus side, this is the most exciting homework you will ever have.) Books and videos can be great resources for learning about Tantra and brushing up on your Tantric techniques. Thanks to modern technology, it is easier than ever to study Tantra in many different media formats. Taking advantage of all the different ways in which you can learn about Tantra can help you achieve ultimate enlightenment.

Choosing Resources That Are Right for You

When considering stocking up on books, videos, and other extra resources to help with your quest for Tantric knowledge, you must first decide which types of material are best for you. Everyone has his or her own individual style when it comes to learning and retaining new material (regardless of the subject), so it is important to tailor your approach to your specific learning style, in order to get the maximum benefit.

Consider Your Interests and Learning Style

There are many long-winded, wordy Tantric texts out there, and they certainly provide a thorough, in-depth examination of Tantra, its roots, and all of the various philosophies and variations. But if you are not a big fan of long reads, these will not be very helpful to you. Instead, you might be better off with an easier-to-read guide featuring short, snappy bursts of information. Maybe even a Tantric magazine article or booklet would be more your style.

Or maybe you are not much of a reader at all. You may be the type of person who learns best by seeing something demonstrated before your very eyes. In this case, videos may be the best bet for you. This can also be a good choice if you would like to be able to show your partner specific techniques or positions that interest you.

Books

Since you are reading this book right now, it probably goes without saying that you understand the value of books in conveying information and important ideas. That is very fortunate, as books can be a huge help to you in your quest for Tantric awareness and enlightenment. Fortunately, there are lots of books about Tantra, written in many different styles and formats. If you scan the sex or relationships shelf of your nearest bookstore or library, you should find a wide variety of choices for your reading pleasure.

Different Books, Different Views

While you have hopefully found this book to be very helpful, it would be impossible for any one book to tell you everything you want to know about Tantra and Tantric sex. So you should make it a point to read as many books on the topic as you can, in order to achieve the greatest level of enlightenment possible. Many books focus on specific aspects of Tantra—its long and rich history, for example, or its emphasis on unity and closeness.

Some books are written from a strictly traditional Tantric viewpoint, stressing the ancient beliefs, while others take more of a modern Neo-Tantric approach. You will probably tend to gravitate toward books that complement your own Tantric approach, although it can be interesting to research other forms of Tantra, as well.

Also, many of the books and e-books out there were written by Tantric teachers and gurus, each of whom has a slightly different viewpoint and system of beliefs. By exposing yourself to a wide range of Tantric thoughts and opinions, you can make a fully informed choice as to which path is right for you.

It can also be interesting to see how these Tantric teachers/authors—while endorsing the same basic philosophy—put their own spin on the subject, adapting it to meet their specific needs and beliefs.

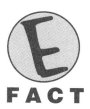

FACT

In a recent survey conducted by MSNBC, 52 percent of women and 41 percent of men said they regularly read magazine articles or books that promise to "put the spark back in your relationship." Bottom line: There are a lot of people out there hoping to find the key to a better sex life in the written word.

Many of the new and popular books on Tantric sex are printed on visually pleasing glossy paper with a lot of romantic and attractive photos and illustrations. In fact, some of these books look more like an art collection catalog than a sex guide. Many people find these types of books more interesting and easier to read, especially because the photos (often featuring couples actually demonstrating the techniques or engaging in the positions) clearly illustrate the material being described in the text.

As the old saying goes, "A picture is worth a thousand words." And this is very true when it comes to sexual instruction in general, and Tantric sex specifically. It is one thing to hear a technique described. It is often far more effective to see a technique demonstrated with your own eyes. By looking at a book with rich artwork and pleasing colors, you will automatically feel a little bit more sensual before you even read a single word.

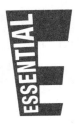

For a great example of a richly illustrated book on Tantric sex that features helpful photos and romantic art, check out *The Art of Tantric Sex,* written by Nitya Lacroix. You will love the book's warm colors and easy-to-read content. Another good choice is *Tantric Love* by Ma Ananda Sarita and Swami Anand Geho.

You can find a list of suggested books and videos in the Resources section at the back of this book. In addition, be sure to check out the online resources listed. Virtually every Tantra Web site features a section where you can order books and other materials.

Videos

While books and other resources can be very helpful, sometimes there is just no substitute for watching techniques demonstrated in action. In many cases, especially with more advanced or complicated positions and techniques, it can often be difficult to envision exactly what they would look like in person. And even the best illustrations can still only provide a two-dimensional view of the material.

Videos allow you to see specific techniques being practiced by real-life people. Even better, you can learn at your own pace, rewinding and replaying segments of particular interest. Not to mention, many of these videos can serve as a great way to get your libido moving, so it can be a good idea to incorporate them into your foreplay routine.

If there are certain techniques or positions you would really like to try, you can also use the videos to show your partner exactly what you have in mind.

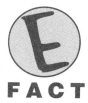

FACT

Adult videos are no small-time operation nowadays. This type of entertainment makes up a $20 billion business in the United States. There are 800 million rentals each year of adult videos and DVDs—and there is plenty of material to choose from, since 11,000 new adult movies are produced each year.

There are tons of adult videos out there that can show you how to spice up your sex life. But there are also an increasing number of videos specifically focused on Tantra and Tantric sex, as well as related topics like the Kama Sutra. These videos and DVDs can be extra special because they often feature erotic scenery, sexy music, and romantic settings. They tend to go the extra mile in setting that special scene and establishing an ambience, as opposed to the stereotypical porn scene where people just go at it on a pool table or in the back of a bus. These videos are also relevant because they often spotlight techniques stressed by Tantra, such as female ejaculation, multiple male orgasms, and sexual massage.

In addition, you may also want to check out some of the videos and DVDs focusing specifically on the Kama Sutra.

However, adult videos in general have really come a long way since the early days of cheesy characters and lame plots (or no plots at all). If you cringe at the thought of watching some big-mustached motorcycle cop "accidentally" encounter a broken-down bus full of horny cheerleaders, take heart. Check out some new adult videos, and you might be pleasantly surprised. Adult film producers are increasingly making an effort to create interesting movies that don't insult viewers' intelligence or rely on dated scenarios. More and more adult videos take the time to set a romantic scene and pay attention to details like background music and scenery.

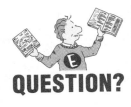

Is there any way to get an adult movie without having to go to a public store?

Yes, you can now rent adult movies from the comfort and privacy of your own home through sites like WantedList.com. It's similar to NetFlix—where you pay for a membership and can rent a few films at a time, keeping them as long as you like—only it offers strictly adult films. Choose from thousands of movies in many different genres.

There is a growing segment of adult videos made for—and by—women. These videos tend to place more of an emphasis on romance and foreplay than the typical porn flick.

Candida Royalle

When it comes to adult videos that cater to women's tastes and erotic preferences, you might say Candida Royalle is the queen. The founder of Femme Productions, Candida has produced numerous erotic films from a woman's unique perspective. As Candida says, "I like to call my Femme movies 'sensually explicit,' or as one viewer described them, the 'Rx for couples.' You'll find them to be less graphic and lacking in the traditional 'money shot,' a staple of most adult films. You'll also find story lines, good original music and real characters of all ages. Counselors often prefer to use my movies in their work with couples because of their woman-friendly approach and what they call positive sexual role modeling."

Candida Royalle has also written several books, including *How to Tell a Naked Man What to Do.* In addition, she helped create the Natural Contours line of vibrators and sexual wellness products.

You can learn more about Candida and view all of her products at *www .candidaroyalle.com*

Video Reluctance

Many people are reluctant to watch adult videos for the first time, for a variety of reasons. For many, it goes back to the same old story—they were taught as children that sex (and anything related to it) is bad or dirty. And for those who were taught that even *thinking* about sex is bad, then surely watching other people have sex must be 100 times worse. Others, especially women, may have always incorrectly assumed that adult movies were strictly for horny old men or perverts.

You Are Not Alone

It can be helpful, if you are reluctant to explore the area of adult films, to realize that lots of "normal" people enjoy these types of movies. You do not have to be weird or sex-crazed to like adult movies, and buying them does not make you unusual or freaky.

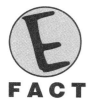

In a recent survey conducted by MSNBC, 37 percent of respondents said they had watched adult movies within the past year in order to help add excitement to their sex lives. Surprisingly, 14 percent said they had taken this a step further and made a tape of their own sexual activities.

Lots of people, including an increasing number of women—from housewives to grandmothers—have become fans of adult films, especially now that it has become so easy to rent or buy them.

You might be surprised to discover that many of your friends and neighbors—yes, even the ones who seem so quiet and reserved—enjoy a racy video on a regular basis. Try broaching the subject in a roundabout way the next time you are enjoying a relaxed get-together with a few close friends. Chances are, a few of them will share their own experiences, if possibly a bit reluctantly at first.

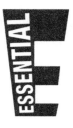

For added convenience and financial savings, you can even buy Tantric and/or mainstream adult DVDs and books that are sold together, sometimes with a bottle of massage oil or some other little surprise thrown in to make the package complete. Check major online adult retailers like Adam & Eve (✎*www.adameve.com*) for package deals.

Self-Consciousness and Body Issues

Some people—especially women—are reluctant to watch adult videos because they fear they will look drab (or fat, old, etc.) when compared to the hot porn stars featured in these videos. They may worry that their partner will wish he were with the knockout in the movie instead.

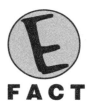

FACT

If you are skittish about watching adult films for the first time in front of your partner, try watching the film by yourself first. This way you won't feel self-conscious about your partner watching your reactions—plus, you can pause the tape at an exciting part to show your partner when the mood is right.

A good way to avoid the self-consciousness issue? Look for amateur tapes, which are available in many adult stores and at lots of online venues. As the name implies, these tapes features scenes involving nonprofessional "stars"—often everyday couples who look like you or people you know. These real people—like all real people—come in all shapes, sizes, and appearances. This can have many positive results for you as a viewer. For one thing, you will get a realistic view of what most people's bodies actually look like—as opposed to the unrealistic porn star body, which has almost always been enhanced by plastic surgery and various other procedures (and further assisted by special lighting and fancy camera tricks). This can be a great reality check—"hey, she has cellulite, too!"—and perhaps even an ego boost—"Wow, my breasts are much perkier than those, and she's younger than me."

More importantly, you are much less likely to feel self-conscious and worry that you will suffer in comparison to the people in these films. You may also learn some new tricks by observing how real people—in the midst of real passion, not the fake on-screen kind—make love in new and exciting ways.

Adjuncts to Workshops

It can be helpful to use books and DVDs in conjunction with Tantra workshops to maximize the benefit of the instructions and information you receive. Many workshops offer related materials such as videos and books for sale at their events. Take advantage of these extras whenever possible. During the workshop itself, it can often be challenging to understand every nugget of information—let alone remembering it all when you get home later. These extra materials can be a valuable help when you are trying to put your newfound knowledge into real-life action.

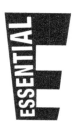

If your partner was unable to attend the workshop with you, having some books or DVDs that tie in with the topic can be a great way to help demonstrate the things you have learned. Bonus: You will get the chance to play "teacher," which your partner may find sexy.

In addition, if the same person or people who taught the workshop also appear on the video, this can be comforting and reassuring. It can almost make you feel like an old friend is there with you, serving as your own personal love coach. This type of personal connection can put you at ease and make you feel more relaxed about watching an adult movie.

Using These Materials to Learn

Without a doubt, adult films (as well as books and other materials) can be fun and pleasurable to watch, purely from an entertainment standpoint.

And you are certainly free to watch as many videos as you like, as often as you like, just for the fun of it. However, from a standpoint of enriching your special relationship with a Tantric approach, you should also view these videos as educational tools.

Your Own In-House Instructor

It can be helpful, especially if you are nervous or embarrassed about watching adult videos, to think of this as an educational experience. This is a homework assignment, part of your education in pursuit of a degree in better sex. Just because the material is not presented in a clinical or boring way does not mean it isn't part of an important learning experience. Think of the people in the video as your own personal sex instructors. Only instead of presenting some long, boring lecture, they are giving you a hands-on (excuse the pun) demonstration on a topic of great personal importance to you.

The video stars are showing you exactly what to do and how to do it. They can also give clues as to how difficult or uncomfortable a certain position may be. Perhaps most importantly, they will show you how to worship your partner's body in exactly the right way, which will be sure to drive them wild.

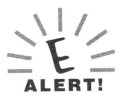

ALERT!

It is important to consider adult books and videos and other materials as instructional guides that help improve and enhance your private relationship with your partner, but never distract from it. Be careful not to become so engrossed in the tapes that your partner feels ignored or neglected. Even the best film is no substitute for a good partner.

Helping Express Your Dislikes

Videos can be useful in helping you show your partner what you like—and, perhaps more importantly, what you *do not* like. In fact, this is a perfect way to convey your sexual dislikes to your partner in a neutral setting where there is no risk of hurt feelings. Think about it: If your partner tries something new in bed that you do not particularly care for, it can be tough to express your reaction in a way that does not hurt your partner's feelings. No matter how you couch it, your partner will most likely take your displeasure as a personal criticism, not just a dislike for that particular move or technique.

However, when you are watching a video and you happen to see something that you do not like (and, thus, that you would like to discourage your partner from attempting), you can simply say something to the effect of, "Hmmm . . . that doesn't seem to be very enjoyable." Or, "That looks interesting, but it really isn't my cup of tea." (Of course, to make it extremely obvious that you do not like what you see, you can always hit the eject button or change the channel.)

This way, you get your point across without any danger of hurting your partner's feelings or appearing critical of his efforts.

Setting Aside the Time Needed

As with anything else worth doing, studying sexual techniques takes time and effort. If you want to brush up on your bedroom skills, you will need to invest some time in your "research"—meaning, reading your books and watching your tapes. This is not something you want to squeeze in on the fly. You really want to be able to concentrate on the material.

It might take some planning and preparation, but you need to set aside some time when you can view your books or videos in privacy, preferably in peace and quiet.

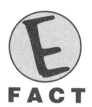

FACT

A typical Tantra video can be an hour long or more. Some adult videos can even run several hours long. Books on Tantra or other sexual topics can easily exceed 200 pages.

Need something quicker for a crash course? Look for a quality adult magazine (choose carefully, as many adult publications contain offensive and overly graphic images).

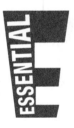

If you have discovered a Tantric video or DVD (or any other kind of adult movie) that you really like, spread the word. Post positive reviews on sites like Amazon.com or the Tantra message boards. You will be doing your fellow Tantrics a favor, as this will make it easier for them to make a good choice.

If you plan to review these materials together with your partner, coordinate your schedules and arrange a "date" for a time when you both will be able to relax and focus on the task at hand. Odds are, this will give you something to look forward to while you are at work or otherwise engaged in your less-pleasurable daily tasks.

This may take some doing, but it will be well worth the effort. Spending some time improving your bedroom techniques and studying "intimate instructional material" with your partner is one of the best investments you can make to strengthen that special bond.

Chapter 18

Sex-ercises

It is no secret that there is a direct corre-lation between your physical condition and your emotional and spiritual well-being. When your body is in good shape, everything else benefits as a result. Even better: When you and your partner get in shape together, you can share a strong bonding experience while also enjoying the sexy new state of each other's bod-ies. Bottom line: You have nothing to lose by stepping up your fitness program (except those love handles).

Getting In Shape Together

It is common knowledge that it is much easier to stick with a fitness routine if you have a "workout buddy" to keep you motivated and serve as your support system. Even better if your workout partner is your spouse or significant other, who can really help encourage you to reach your fitness goals. If you are not feeling particularly enthusiastic during a workout, your partner can distract you by discussing various events in your life—or even by whispering naughty "sweet nothings" in your ear. Not to mention, embarking on this fitness program together can be a great bonding experience that encourages teamwork in all aspects of your relationship. Plus, you are bound to get turned on as you watch each other's bodies get tighter and firmer.

Nancy Kennedy, cofounder of Kennedy Strom Fitness in Los Angeles, says there is a definite connection between physical fitness and sexual fulfillment. "Working out increases your libido as you wake your body up," she says. "You feel your body. It is not numb. You walk taller and are more aware of your muscles and how they feel and where they are. All of this also builds confidence, which increases your sex drive. Increasing blood flow throughout the body will also increase arousal."

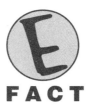

FACT

Taoists and other ancient people believed you could tell a lot about people's sexual prowess and genital characteristics by studying their appearance. For example, someone with a lot of hair on his face and body was thought to have a strong sex drive. Men with long noses were assumed to be well endowed, as were men with long fingers.

And getting in shape with your partner is bound to have a positive impact on your relationship, Kennedy says. "Working out together is another way to spice up your sex life. Not only do you feel the benefits like heightened awareness but watching each other lift, sweat, and strain can be very stimulating. Touching each other and assisting with lifts really brings two people closer. You can walk into the gym mad at your partner and walk out in love and ready to go. . . !"

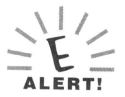

If you embark on a workout routine with your partner, be very selective about any "constructive criticism" you offer with regard to their effort or performance. If you make your partner self-conscious, the negative fallout will quickly erase any benefits you may have gained from this joint activity.

Choosing a Good Joint Fitness Program

Now that you have decided to embark on a fitness program together and reap some of these benefits, you should put some thought into the specific type of program that will work best for both of you. Consider your individual fitness levels and physical abilities. This is especially important if there is a great disparity between your fitness level and that of your partner. You want to choose activities that will challenge you, of course, but if one partner finds it impossible to keep up, they will quickly become discouraged and frustrated, which will cause tension in the relationship.

This is why it can be a good idea to select a program that allows for flexibility and can be tailored to each of your individual fitness levels. A program involving weights, for example, is a good choice because you can easily adjust the weight involved to accommodate the person's abilities.

It can be a good idea to choose activities related to things you both enjoy. If you are both snow lovers, for example, look into getting a season pass at the closest ski resort. (Bonus: After hitting the slopes, you can enjoy warming each other up while cuddling in front of the fire in the ski lodge.) Love to get your groove on and dance the night away? See if there are any dance classes for couples in your area.

It is even better if you can find an activity that reminds you of a special experience or shared memory that evokes positive feelings for both of you. Remember that special island getaway where you went snorkeling before making love on the beach? Perhaps you can recapture that romantic feeling by joining a swimming program—or maybe even by learning how to scuba dive together. Perhaps you can even go on a second honeymoon that involves some kind of outdoor adventure or enjoyable physical activities.

Visualization

As with many parts of Tantra, visualization is important when it comes to getting in better shape. Envision your body getting stronger and slimmer. Picture yourself healthier and leaner than you have been in ages. Imagine how much longer you will be able to sustain sexual encounters once you have increased your strength and stamina.

Visualize yourself becoming more powerful and enjoying greater control over your body during sex. Envision all the extra powerful sexual energy you will have once you have built your body into an efficient physical machine. Better yet, think about how this sexual power will then be doubled if you and your partner both become stronger physically.

Picture your entire body—and your chakras—becoming re-energized from this infusion of strong sexual energy. It will be like fuel that recharges your entire body and soul. This energy will course through your inner flute, firing up all of your chakras and helping you achieve a higher state of consciousness. You will be a strong supreme being, an all-powerful god or goddess.

Kegel Exercises

One important type of routine you can do to improve your sex life is called Kegel exercises. PC (pubococcygeal) muscle exercises (also known as Kegel exercises) help strengthen the muscles in your pelvic region. Kegel exercises are known by many different names. In addition to the term *PC exercises*, these moves are sometimes also called *pelvic floor exercisers*, *pelvic toners*, or *PC trainers*. These exercises stimulate blood flow to the pelvic area and give you greater control over all of the individual muscles in that region. This is a good thing for many reasons, but the most obvious benefit is that it helps women maintain a tighter grip on the penis during sex. Their partners are often amazed at the woman's renewed "tightness"—sometimes saying it feels like having sex with a virgin.

Many people mistakenly believe Kegels are only for women. On the contrary, men can benefit from practicing these exercises as well. Strengthening these muscles can help men maintain stronger, longer-lasting erections.

And for women, the benefits include heightened sensation during sex, more powerful orgasms, and better overall pelvic conditioning and control. On a less exciting but just as important note, strengthening your pelvic floor and the associated muscles can also help prevent problems such as urinary incontinence, uterine prolapse, and bladder problems. All in all, it is a win-win situation.

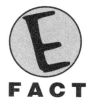

FACT

Kegel exercises were introduced to Western medicine by a gynecologist and obstetrician named Dr. Arnold Kegel in the 1940s. He originally recommended them to help older woman fight incontinence, and also to help women regain vaginal strength and tightness after childbirth. But it didn't take long for women to realize that these exercises could also greatly improve their sex lives.

These exercises are simple to do—and can be done almost anywhere, at any time. (However, in the beginning, it's usually best to do them in the privacy of your home while sitting on the bed or floor. You might also try putting a pillow or rolled-up towel underneath you, as some people find that the slight pressure on their pelvic floor makes it easier for them to get accustomed to doing these exercises.) You just contract your pelvic muscles, as if you were trying to stop a flow of urine. Hold this contraction for a second, then release. Be sure to let your muscles relax fully between each repetition. Some people like to do 100 or more Kegels a day.

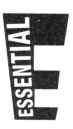

It is important to coordinate your breathing when doing Kegel exercises. Inhale while contracting, hold your breath while clenching, and then exhale when releasing. Most likely, you will find that your breathing falls into line naturally as you do these routines.

Advanced Kegels

Once you have mastered the basic Kegel, you can take things to the next level and step it up to something a bit more challenging. Try holding the "contracted" position longer—maybe while inhaling and exhaling without releasing the hold. Or try to relax your muscles very slowly and gradually, rather than in one swift movement. You should also vary between fast, intense Kegels and slow, more sustained moves. This will target different muscles in that area and ensure that you strengthen the entire muscle group.

Isolate the Individual Muscles

After you have been doing this for a while and have mastered the basic Kegel, you will probably have a whole new outlook on the muscles in your pelvic region. At first, you probably thought there was just one big muscle that controlled the whole operation down there. If that were the case, doing the Kegel exercises regularly was probably a valuable learning experience for you. By this point, you should have realized that the pelvic region involves not just one muscle, but several different groups of muscles, each of which work independently and perform different functions.

As you strengthen your pelvic floor and become adept at doing Kegels, you will also learn how to isolate each individual group of pelvic muscles. By isolating each individual muscle or group of muscles, you can reap the maximum rewards from these exercises. Not only will you be able to strengthen these muscles more efficiently, but you will learn how to identify and control each muscle individually. As a result, you will be able to contract and flex these muscles in ways you never could before—making for some exciting new sensations during sexual encounters. Most likely, these moves will not go unnoticed by your partner, who will also reap the rewards of your newfound mastery of the PC muscles. This is especially true in the case of men, who often enjoy displaying their pelvic mastery by demonstrating their ability to control the movement of their penis in new and improved ways.

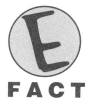

Women can maximize the benefits of these exercises by purchasing a Kegel egg (also called a *vaginal strengthening egg*). The Kegelmaster is another "toy" that is helpful for this purpose. Or, just about any sex toy will do. Simply tense your PC muscles as you try to remove it, doing your best to resist the pulling action and trying to hold the toy in.

The Elevator

A common type of advanced Kegel routine is known as "the Elevator." You will only be able to attempt this after you have totally mastered the basic Kegel. You will contract your pelvic muscles slowly. Imagine they are an elevator. When the elevator is on the first floor, you are in a relaxed state. Then slowly start trying to pull the elevator up to the first floor by contracting the first set of muscles. Move on to the second floor, the third, and so on. When you reach the top floor and have contracted all of your pelvic muscles, hold that state for a moment. Then slowly release, bringing the elevator back down, one floor at a time.

Pulsing

Another advanced variation of the Kegel is called pulsing or fluttering. This is where you quickly tighten and release the PC muscle in a pulsating rhythm over several seconds. For a real challenge, try doing a pulsating move while you are on the "top floor" of your elevator technique.

Pompoir

Strengthening your pelvic muscles through Kegel exercises will improve your sex life in many ways. One of the major benefits is that it will allow you to master the art of pompoir, which is a great little trick to have in your sexual arsenal. Pompoir is the ancient art of "milking" the lingam (penis) of your partner by tightly squeezing your PC muscles during intercourse. This was initially a top-secret practice that was only taught to a select few women—mainly, the consorts of royalty. However, word soon spread that this technique could send male lovers through the roof, so soon many women wanted to learn this trick.

Here is a trick to help you perform the pompoir technique: While having sex, contract your PC muscles rapidly to "milk" or "pump" your lover's penis. Try this out during sex without informing your lover beforehand. Watch his eyes light up at this exciting surprise! Experimentation is important here. Pompoir creates different sensations depending on which position you are in. You can also vary the experience by changing the speed or intensity of your PC contractions. Ask your partner which ways feel more pleasurable for him.

Dance and Movement

Dancing is a great form of exercise. You can burn off a ton of calories, and really get quite a workout—especially if you dance to some really fast music. The best part? It doesn't feel like exercise!

Dancing, especially at a fast pace, can recharge your entire body. It gets your blood pumping quickly and sends lots of endorphins rushing to your brain. In fact, many people claim they reach states similar to an orgasmic high during fast-paced dance sessions. Dancing offers lots of physical benefits such as stronger muscles, improved coordination, and the physical effects of aerobic exercises.

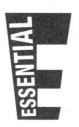

Dancing can be an extremely effective form of exercise. Aerobic (high intensity) dancing can work off more than 500 calories in an hour. Now that's a workout! Even slower-paced forms of dance like ballroom dancing can burn more than 200 calories an hour. So not only can dancing make you feel sexier, but you will look sexier, as well.

But dance can be especially great as an exercise that will help improve your love life. From a physical standpoint, it helps tone your muscles and improve your flexibility. Needless to say, this can come in handy in the bedroom. In addition, by learning to move your body in a rhythmic way, you will feel more comfortable moving it a similar way during sexual encounters. You will grow more comfortable in your own skin, and you won't feel as self-conscious about moving your body.

You will also become more aware of your body and will start to develop your own natural sense of rhythm and control over your body's movements. Plus, people—especially women—tend to feel sexier when they are dancing. This is especially true if you have a male admirer (or several) appreciatively enjoying your moves. Often, men will get extremely turned on just by watching their partner dance, especially if she is uninhibited and is obviously enjoying herself. This positive attention can also be a great boost to the ego and give you a burst of self-confidence that will translate into more confidence and assertiveness during sex.

Dancing is great from a relationship angle, too. Many couples enjoy dancing together and find the closeness of slow dancing to be very romantic. This can be a great warm-up activity to enjoy as part of your foreplay ritual. Also, by dancing together regularly, you can learn how to get your individual rhythms in sync, which can also be an advantage in the bedroom.

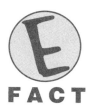

FACT

Dancing can be an extremely erotic and arousing act, so it can be a good idea to include this as part of your foreplay routine. Practice a particularly sensual type of dance—like belly dancing or maybe even a striptease routine—and surprise your partner with a private show. There are DVDs available that can show you how to perform a sexy dance routine.

Pelvic Thrusts

Pelvic thrusting is an integral part of sexual activity. It can also be challenging and exhausting, especially if you are not in shape or are out of practice. It doesn't help matters that many people also have a natural tendency to move their pelvis in a stilted or hesitant manner. For these people, it takes an effort to learn how to loosen up and move their pelvic area more freely. That is why it is important to practice pelvic thrusting on a regular basis. Fortunately, this can be lots of fun!

Start by putting on some upbeat, fast-paced music that will really make you want to start moving. Begin by thrusting your hips from front to back while standing up, starting out slowly. Concentrate on the movement, and try to isolate it just to your pelvic area—moving only your hips, while keeping your upper body as still and steady as possible. Focus on allowing your body to move in a loose, relaxed way. Because the same repeated type of thrusting can get boring after a while, you should also work on developing several different types of thrusting patterns. Try a slow, rhythmic pattern, a fast, frantic pattern, and perhaps a sensual type of thrusting similar to a belly dancer's movements. Having a whole repertoire of thrusting moves will help you vary your lovemaking experiences and create lots of different sensations and experiences that you and your partner will both enjoy. Thrusting preferences can vary widely from one person (and couple) to another. Some women find hard, quick thrusting to be uncomfortable—perhaps even painful—especially for extended periods of time. Plus, slow thrusting can help build the excitement and anticipation, kind of like a teaser before the real action gets started. On the other hand, there are people who like their thrusting fast and furious, all the time. Ideally, you and your partner are on the same page with your thrusting preferences. If not, you can compromise by incorporating the types of thrusting each of you prefers into your overall sexual routine.

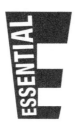

Different types and speeds of pelvic thrusting stimulate specific parts of the body in different ways. One type of thrusting may be better for G-spot stimulation, while another is more conducive to clitoral orgasms. Experiment with different types of thrusting to learn the specific sensations and results you get from each.

Pelvic Lifts

Pelvic lifts are similar to pelvic thrusts, but you practice them while lying on the floor. This makes sense because, after all, you will often be lying down while doing pelvic thrusting during sex. To practice pelvic lifts, you simply lie on your back with your knees bent while lifting your hips up and down off the floor. When you lift your hips up, try to hold them in that position for several seconds to really strengthen your muscles. Bonus: When you do this, you will naturally contract your abdominal muscles, basically doing a "crunch" exercise, so you get a great ab workout in the process.

Practicing Pelvic Thrusts as a Couple

It can be exciting (and entertaining) to practice pelvic thrusts together with your partner. Pay attention to how your partner moves, and how this differs from or complements your own natural movements. This will allow you to synchronize your thrusting techniques and perfect your thrusting patterns in unison. Later during lovemaking you will probably find that you automatically fall into this synchronized pattern right away. Watching each other doing all of this pelvic thrusting can be a big turn-on, so pelvic thrusting practice often ends up becoming a form of foreplay.

Chapter 19

Especially for Her

In Tantra, the woman is put on a pedestal. She is seen as a goddess, the center of the universe. In traditional Tantra, the woman was thought to have godly powers because of her ability to create life and give birth. All women were viewed as likenesses of Shakti, a pure and positive energy force. Every woman was believed to embody the spirit of a goddess, and was to be revered and worshipped.

Women as Goddesses

Tantra views all female human beings as goddesses, born of the earth and the sea. Women are seen as a powerful female energy force, creatures who embody all of the positive aspects of femininity. Women are believed to be in a divine state from the moment of their birth and throughout their entire lives. This status of a goddess is not related to status, class, race, or ethnicity. All women—rich or poor, married or single, young or old—are viewed as goddesses and should be treated that way.

Among other things, this means that Tantric teachings forbid a man from raising his hand to any woman, acting disrespectfully toward her, or mistreating her in any way. "Women's lib" was not an issue, as women were perceived to be equals (if not superiors) to men. This was an interesting paradox: Although admired for being the "softer" beings, women actually wielded the stronger power—just in a less obvious way.

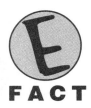

FACT

It is well known that ancient civilizations placed great importance on worshipping gods in female form. These ancient people viewed goddesses as the source of life and nurturer of all living things. It is said that Cleopatra considered herself to be a goddess in human form. Most historians believe goddess worship peaked at least 5,000 years ago.

Like all goddesses, a woman is an all-powerful being, which is reflected in the many important roles she performs: mother, sister, lover, partner, friend, nurturer, giver of life.

Famous Goddesses

There are many well-known goddesses in history and mythology. Eve is seen by many to have been the very first goddess to walk the earth. Perhaps the most famous goddesses are those of Greek and Roman origins, such as Venus, Nike, Aphrodite, and the Muses. Although not officially bestowed with a goddess title, Mary (mother of Christ) is also seen by many as an ultimate goddess figure.

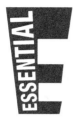

Isis is an important Egyptian goddess because she was a symbol of love, sexuality, and healing. According to legend, Isis differed from most goddesses because she mingled with the mortal people, teaching women homemaking arts like cooking and sewing. She continues to be viewed as the ultimate embodiment of womanhood and femininity.

Hindu goddesses include Lakshmi, the goddess of good fortune and prosperity; Durga, the warrior goddess; and Kali, who symbolizes death and female empowerment and the transcendent aspects of sex.

Treat Her Like the Goddess She Is

In Tantric terms, the idea of viewing your female partner as a goddess refers to treating her with the honor, respect, and reverence that you would for any divine being.

You would never want to mistreat her, disrespect her, or cause her harm in any way. You should aim to please her in every way possible.

Worship Her Sexually

With regard to her body, you should worship it and treat it with reverence and total respect. Your ultimate goal should be to please her and lavish glorious worship upon her body. Her pleasure and satisfaction should be your top priority. Only once she is satisfied can you pursue your own physical pleasure.

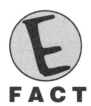

FACT

In modern Tantra environments, the term *goddess* is often used to refer to a woman who provides guidance and instruction (often in private one-on-one settings) to people who wish to learn about Tantra and explore Tantric ideas and practices.

Important: A man should never enter or touch a woman's sacred space without first asking permission. While her thighs may lead to the "gates of heaven," this is not a destination that is automatically open and accessible all of the time. And you should never forget that important rule or take the privilege of being allowed near her sacred space for granted. You must be given an access pass, one that is usually not given casually. And this is true whether this is your first time together or your thousandth. No matter how long she has been your partner, you should never take her for granted or treat her any less respectfully than you did when you were first dating.

Outside of the Bedroom

Although worshipping her during sensual encounters is important, you should not limit your reverence and adulation to the times before and during lovemaking. If you do make this mistake, you will risk looking like a stereotypical male: only being nice to the woman until you get what you want. This is definitely not a good image to present.

Instead, you should be in a state of constant worship and reverence. It is important to show love and respect for your goddess every hour of every day. You must demonstrate this by your words and actions. Make sure to always treat her with kindness and respect and to constantly show her how special she is to you. Give her little treats and gifts out of the blue, for no specific reason. Surprise her with a romantic evening or an exciting getaway just to show her how excited you are to be with her and how much you enjoy her company.

Treat Yourself as the Goddess You Are

Ideally, your partner and others around you will treat you as the goddess you are, and lavish you with the reverence and praise you should rightfully expect. However, don't feel like you need to sit around waiting for someone else to treat you like a goddess. Feel free to take matters into your own hands and enjoy some well-deserved self-indulgence. Unfortunately, for many women, this does not come naturally. Women are taught from an early age to take care of others, so it can often feel indulgent or selfish to take care of yourself. Ignore those thoughts. Keep reminding yourself that you are a divine goddess worthy of life's pleasures.

Bring Out Your Inner Goddess

In traditional Tantric teachings, women were taught the importance of recognizing and nurturing their inner goddess. Women were encouraged to seek their internal goddess powers and embrace them. Only then, it was believed, could the woman seek (and hopefully attain) a transcendental union with her partner. That was also the only way the woman could attain sexual freedom and psychological and emotional healing and growth.

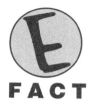

FACT

Want to brush up on your goddess skills? Author Laurie Sue Brockway brings the ancient wisdom of the goddess down to earth for modern women in her book, *A Goddess Is a Girl's Best Friend: A Divine Guide to Finding Love, Success and Happiness.*

A big part of nurturing your inner goddess is recognizing your incredible value and worth. This may not come naturally to women, who are often accustomed to putting themselves and their own needs and desires last. It may take some conscious effort on your part, but you must learn to put yourself first sometimes. First and foremost, guard your health and well-being and make your health needs a top priority. Take the time to exercise, meditate, and do everything else in your power to maintain a healthy lifestyle.

You should also pamper your inner goddess by allowing yourself some well-deserved indulgences. This can be anything from weekly pedicures to a spa retreat with friends.

If you feel selfish indulging yourself, remember that everyone around you will benefit if you are content and feel spiritually nurtured. When you feel good inside, your relationships will reap the benefits. So if not for your own sake, do it for those around you who want to see you happy and who will enjoy the benefits of your joyful state of mind.

Help Is Available

If you need help recognizing and invoking your inner goddess, you are in luck. There are numerous Tantric workshops and events dedicated solely to this topic. For example, a group of female Tantra teachers present frequent workshops called "Embracing the Goddess Within." (For details, visit *www.tantraforwomen.com.*)

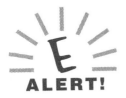

ALERT!

If a female suffers major physical or emotional trauma at an early age (especially if it involves sexual abuse), it is believed that her inner goddess may retreat or hide, leading to fear or avoid sex later on. As a result, it would be important for the woman to make a special effort to bring out the goddess hiding within her.

Set the Stage

Sometimes when you are trying to evoke your inner goddess, it can help if you have the proper environment. Set up a special romantic area for your intimate encounters. If you like, you can even create a little "altar"—not in the religious sense, but a special area dedicated solely to the worship of your goddess spirit. This can also be an important part of your sacred space, where your partner can worship at your feet. Adorn your altar with meaningful mementos, perhaps pictures of yourself, your partner, and other loved ones. Add little meaningful romantic touches, such as souvenirs from romantic getaways with your partner. Place a radio nearby for some soothing music to help set the proper mood. For a finishing touch, adorn your altar with flowers and aromatic candles.

The Art of Dressing

It is much easier to feel like a goddess (and be treated like one) if you look the part. And adorning yourself in proper goddess attire is a big step in the right direction.

What exactly should your perfect goddess outfit look like? That is totally up to you. There is no "standard issue" goddess uniform. The most important thing is wearing something that makes you feel sexy and luxurious (and, ideally, at least moderately comfortable—although, as every woman knows, sometime you need to sacrifice a little comfort for the sake of sexiness).

Many women find it easier to get into the "goddess" state of mind when dressed up in goddesslike garments. So experiment with some ensembles befitting a goddess of ultimate stature: flowing robes, luxurious scarves, romantic gowns in silk or other rich materials. If necessary, start out by telling yourself you are playing a part. You may initially begin just pretending to be a goddess, but soon you will feel the part and realize you truly are a real-life goddess. Make-believe will become a satisfying reality.

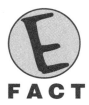

FACT

The West Bengal area of India is one of the most active areas for goddess worship. This region has a long and rich legacy of worshipping goddesses, a tradition that still continues today. For the people of this region, the highlight of each year centers around annual holidays that celebrate specific goddesses—occasions marked by elaborate rituals complete with fireworks, parades, and loud celebrations.

For the full divine effect, you can go for the total goddess image and put your hair in an upsweep or long flowing curls, with a strategically placed flower or two. Add some sparkling jewels and sexy makeup to round out the look.

Become Even More Open and Orgasmic

Perhaps the ultimate celebration of your goddess powers occurs in the form of an orgasm. This is when you truly achieve a higher state of being and transcend into a goddess state.

This may sound strange, but many women simply are not good at receiving pleasure. It is not an automatic thing, and it may not feel natural at first. Women by nature are caretakers, taught from an early age to attend to everyone else's needs. This is especially true when it comes to husbands and partners. Many women are so focused on pleasing their partners that they neglect their own needs. Instead they focus on doing whatever their partner wants and making sure he is satisfied. In the end, women end up feeling frustrated and unfulfilled, but they don't know how to prevent this.

The solution is simple, at least on paper. You need to recognize your needs and give yourself permission to fulfill your desires. This pleasure is rightfully yours, well deserved, and befitting your status as a goddess. Remind yourself that you do not need to be the caretaker and provider of pleasure all of the time. Sometimes it is okay to be "selfish" sexually and allow your partner to please you, possibly without any reciprocation on your part. This will actually in turn heighten your partner's pleasure, because most men become aroused by pleasing their woman. If it helps, think of it as doing him a favor by granting him the privilege of pleasuring you. Besides, you will "even the score" by treating him to a night of total indulgence when it is his turn.

Roadblocks to Orgasm

Unfortunately, even though orgasm is a very natural process, many women have great difficulty reaching this point. They get sidetracked and thrown off track by physical, emotional, and mental obstacles. It is imperative for women to learn how to get rid of these obstacles, or heal any existing wounds, in order to pursue their destined orgasmic state.

The first and most important step is to open yourself up to the experience of total satisfaction. Many women falsely believe they are being open and receptive to this experience, when in fact they have put up various roadblocks.

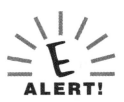
ALERT!

If you are allowing your mind to wander during sex, and you are thinking about whether your thighs look big, whether you are making any strange noises—or even if you forgot to drop off the dry cleaning earlier today—you are blocking the road to orgasm by making yourself mentally distracted. This is a time when you need full concentration and focus.

One major (and common) obstacle: expecting your partner(s) to *give* you an orgasm. This is a lot of pressure to put on your partner, and the sexual experience. Your partner does not give you an orgasm, although he may greatly help accelerate the process. But this cannot happen unless you allow yourself to receive this help, by opening yourself up to the idea and welcoming the climax, allowing orgasm to happen.

Another roadblock to orgasm is thinking too much. Many women have trouble freeing their minds during sex and allowing themselves to just *feel* without overanalyzing the situation. Instead, they start obsessing about their long-established beliefs that sex is dirty or bad. Talk about a mood killer! This will immediately cause them to tense up and block the road to bliss, even if they don't consciously realize it.

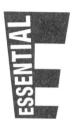

A man can help his female partner open herself up to orgasm by providing lots of encouragement and support throughout the entire intimate encounter. He should remind her repeatedly how excited he gets by seeing her enjoying pleasure and by watching her give in to the sensations freely and without inhibitions.

Female Ejaculation

While on the topic of women and orgasm, this would probably be a good place to discuss the phenomenon of female ejaculation. This is actually a controversial subject, with many people believing it does not exist at all. People in this doubting camp believe that this "ejaculatory fluid" is actually urine that is released involuntary during sex. However, traditional Taoists and Tantrics not only believed in female ejaculation, they viewed it with a kind of reverence, as a special act.

Female ejaculation refers to the release of a noticeable amount of fluid by a woman during orgasm. Even among people who believe in female ejaculation, there is much debate and differing opinions on things like what exactly is contained in the fluid, where it comes from, and whether every woman has the ability to experience ejaculation. It is usually thought that female ejaculation is most likely to occur as a result of G-spot stimulation.

Recent research seems to support the theory that most women do indeed release this fluid during an orgasm—although they might not realize it because the fluid is usually a very small amount and (despite what may be portrayed in some adult films) generally does not come gushing out with incredible force.

Enhancing Her Pleasure

No matter how exciting, a sexual encounter is not considered totally successful unless both parties have achieved the ultimate level of pleasure. Although women can sometimes seem difficult to satisfy, there are many things you as man can do to enhance your female partner's pleasure.

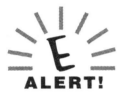

ALERT!

While it can take effort to enhance her pleasure, never think of this as a job or a chore. This is a privilege and you should revel in the opportunity to help your partner achieve satisfied bliss. Plus, keep in mind, the more turned-on and satisfied she is, the more exciting the experience is likely to be for you.

Perhaps the most important thing you can do to enhance her pleasure is to be a totally receptive and giving partner. Encourage her to tell you her wants, needs, and desires—and make sure your reactions are positive and nonjudgmental. Communicate with her, ask a lot of questions, and be a good listener. Let her know that her pleasure is your top priority.

From a physical standpoint, you can enhance her pleasure by taking things slow and let her (and her body) set the pace. Rushing things before she is mentally or physically ready can kill the mood—and can also be physically uncomfortable for a woman, whose body must be physically prepared for sexual union.

Worship her entire body, but during the height of lovemaking, pay special attention to the clitoris. When it comes to her physical pleasure, the clitoris is the heart of the operation. Practice your technique for "polishing the pearl" so you can pleasure her orally. You should also be receptive to the idea of using sex toys (especially those designed for clitoral stimulation) to help her reach orgasm. If she doesn't suggest it, you can carefully broach the topic—but tread carefully, and never exert pressure on her to try anything before she is ready. You can also encourage her to try sexual creams or gels designed to heighten female arousal.

In addition, you can be sure to spend lots of time in positions that are known to provide maximum female pleasure, such as the rear-entry positions and any others that she particularly favors.

Increasing Libido

For many women, the biggest major roadblock to sexual pleasure is a lagging libido. Many women complain that they often just do not feel "in the mood." This is common, especially for today's busy woman, who is often juggling a career, kids, partner, and many other responsibilities. Understandably so, the woman may feel so stressed or tired that sex is the last thing on her mind.

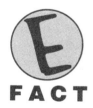

FACT

A low sex drive is a common problem in American women. The American Medical Association has estimated that several million U.S. women suffer from what doctors prefer to call "female sexual arousal disorder," or "FSAD." That's a fancy way of saying their libido is in need of life support.

The first step to solving this problem is to be a helpful and supportive partner. Help around the house, be an active co-parent, and do whatever else you can to help shoulder the responsibilities and take a little bit of stress off her mind. Encourage her to relax and take some time to de-stress at the end of the day. If necessary, have the grandparents take the kids for the night (or hire a sitter and whisk your woman off to some peaceful getaway). Just getting some rest and escaping from the constant pressures of everyday life can be a big libido boost for many women.

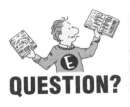

QUESTION?

Are there other causes for a low sex drive besides stress?
Many medical conditions can affect your sex drive—including quite a few that are easily fixed. For women, hormonal imbalances are a common culprit. If you make an active effort to reduce your daily stress and your libido is still lacking, it may be time to consult a doctor. In addition, if you are taking any medications, read the side effects carefully, as this is a common source of sexual problems.

If the libido still is not up to par, it can be helpful to engage in some slow foreplay, without any expectations that intercourse will follow. Often, eliminating this pressure to perform will help the woman relax, and hopefully the foreplay will leave her so aroused that she will in fact feel the urge to make love.

You can also try some of the "libido creams" and other sexual products designed to arouse a woman and stimulate her libido. However, you should use these with caution. Try a very small amount at first, until you can evaluate how they work. Some women find these products to be annoying or find that they cause a sensation that is too intense for sensitive areas.

If you suspect that some past trauma or emotional problems are contributing to your low sex drive, a consultation with a therapist or psychologist might prove very helpful.

Chapter 20

Especially for Him

While the woman has a special place in Tantra, the man is of course very important, as well. In addition to pleasing and honoring the goddess, men were highly regarded for their own special qualities. Men were traditionally worshipped for their strength and power. They were also looked upon to be leaders and to make wise decisions. They were expected to be the voice of authority and to be providers and protectors for their families.

Men as Gods

Just as Tantra views women as goddesses, so too are men viewed as powerful godlike beings. While the same basic tenets apply—he should be worshipped, adored, and revered—there are some distinct differences.

Treating Him as God

Treating your man as a god is in many ways similar to the ways in which he should treat you as a goddess. You should respect and honor him and treat his body as a sacred instrument. You should also strive to please him, and—in deference to his manhood—appreciate his masculinity and virility. While you certainly should not be totally submissive and allow yourself to be controlled, it is okay (and, in fact, probably encouraged) for you to occasional let him "call the shots" and defer to his wishes and decisions.

Famous Gods

There are two types of famous gods: the religious kind, and those of mythology. (It is important to note, though, that what today is considered mythology—such as the worship of ancient Greek gods—was considered a religion by the people of that time period who practiced it.) Under the religious heading, there is God in the Christian form, Allah, Yahweh, Buddha, and others. Egyptians, meanwhile, believed their pharaohs were immortal and would become gods after their earthly deaths. Tantrics, of course, revered the god Shiva.

When discussing the mythical type of god, probably the most famous is Zeus. Zeus was considered the "head honcho" of the Greek gods. He was believed to rule the heavens and have hierarchy above all of the other gods. He was worshipped for his awesome power, which was often symbolized by a lightning bolt. Another famous god was Zeus's brother Hades, who ruled over the underworld. You might say he was the direct opposite of Zeus. Hades was often feared because he symbolized death, as well as negative characteristics like anger and greed.

Gods Versus Goddesses

While goddesses were believed to have been created from the earth and sea, gods were believed to have their roots in the sun. Along those lines, they are respected for being strong and full of powerful energy, like Zeus and his lightning bolts.

Tantrics believed that the man's responsibility as a god was to live an honest and ethical life. Whereas the goddess must nurture and sustain, the god must protect and lead. He must be a source of strength, wisdom, and power. He was also expected to be the leader of the family, and possibly an authority figure for the community.

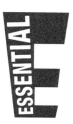

Although a man/god is expected to be masculine and strong, he should also not be afraid to express his "softer side." Tantrics believe a man should feel free to show his vulnerability and sensitivity. After all, one basic tenet of Tantra is that everyone has a yin and yang—both a feminine and masculine side.

Gods and goddesses both play specific roles when it comes to Tantra. Neither is more important than the other, and in fact, they cannot exist independently without the other. For cosmic harmony, both the god and goddess must exist together in a perfect union. They must join together to establish the perfect balance, the yin and yang that leads to a state of bliss and balance.

Ejaculation Mastery

A major tenet in Tantric beliefs is the importance of ejaculation mastery. Many ancient gurus believed ejaculation was a waste of vital life energy, so men were taught to condition themselves to preserve their seminal fluid and to release it as infrequently as possible. This was because of the great drain on physical energy and vital force when a man ejaculates. It was also believed that men should instead use that energy as fuel for awakening the higher chakra centers and thus to move on to enlightenment.

As a result, traditional Tantric men became experts at controlling (and avoiding) ejaculation. Sometimes this involved considerable effort or complicated processes. One Tantric text describes a specific elaborate pattern of strokes of movements that, if the man followed them exactly, were said to prevent him from reaching a level of excitement that would allow ejaculation to occur. Other techniques were extremely simple, such as pressing the tongue against the roof of the mouth.

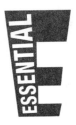

Although Chinese Taoism (and, to a lesser extent, Tantra) dictated strict orgasm and ejaculation control for men, the instruction for women was just the opposite. Women were encouraged to have frequent and multiple orgasms, including the secretion of female ejaculate, if possible. This was believed to be a vital substance from which her partner could derive energy and power.

Men would also delay orgasm in order to prolong the sexual union until they were certain they had pleased their goddess (satisfied their female partner). It was also commonly believed that keeping his penis inside the woman for as long as possible without ejaculating enabled the man to absorb some of the woman's vital life juices and powerful energy.

Today, there is some division on the importance of ejaculation (or avoidance of ejaculation). Some still believe it is important to completely avoid ejaculation, while others disagree. Men understand that they are not going to "run out" of seminal fluid. However, it is still considered important to delay the orgasm as long as possible, in order to allow for a long, satisfying sexual encounter.

The easiest and most common way to avoid ejaculation is simply the start-and-stop technique. Just like it sounds, with this technique the man participates in sex as usual, until he gets to the point where he feels he is about to ejaculate. He then stops completely, and perhaps even squeezes or puts pressure on his penis to help the urge to ejaculate subside a bit. Once the urge to ejaculate has receded somewhat, the man can then proceed with the lovemaking process. He can continue with this start/stop pattern until he is ready to ejaculate (or if it becomes uncomfortable), at which point he should allow himself the release.

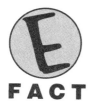

FACT

Early Tao writings describe how a man could delay ejaculation by closing his mouth, opening his eyes wide, and regulating his breathing. It is also suggested that he press a specific point near his right breast, which was believed to be connected with semen retention.

Other techniques that are said to sometimes help in delaying a man's orgasm include pressing on the perineum (spot between scrotum and anus) or pulling gently on the testicle right before orgasm is about to occur. Both of these techniques should be performed carefully and gently, to avoid pain or injury.

Male Multiple Orgasm

Most people believe that women are the only ones who can have multiple orgasms. They believe that with men it is generally a one-shot deal. That is not true at all. Neo-Tantra encourages men to pursue multiple orgasms and teaches techniques to help them achieve that goal.

Men are fully capable of having multiple orgasms, although this is often much easier for young men (in their late teens and twenties) and becomes more difficult as they get older. A younger man can often recover quite quickly from an ejaculatory orgasm and go on to have another ejaculatory orgasm during the same session of lovemaking, while older men find this much more difficult to do—primarily because they have lower testosterone levels. However, younger men can find it more difficult to delay ejaculation and thus build a high enough sexual charge to have one energy-based orgasm, let alone a number of them. Older men, on the other hand, can usually last longer along the way to ejaculation (again because testosterone is lower) and thus can build their charge toward nonejaculatory orgasm.

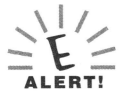

ALERT!

The key to understanding male multiple orgasms is realizing that orgasm and ejaculation are two totally different processes. With a multiple orgasm, the man climaxes several times, but only ejaculates once (if at all). Men are generally unable to ejaculate more than once within a very short time period.

Generally, the "PC squeeze" is considered the most effective way to achieve multiple orgasms by allowing a man to climax without ejaculating. Immediately before the point of climax, a man should squeeze his PC muscles tightly (while also ceasing all stimulation of the penis) until the peak passes. This will probably take some practice, which is usually best done during masturbation.

The Nine Types of Male Movement

In the Kama Sutra, you learn about the nine types of genital movements made by a man. By mastering these basic moves (and using them in creative combinations), the man can come up with his own distinctive sexual techniques.

- **Forward movement:** moving penis forward, directly into the vagina
- **Piercing:** Woman lowers her yoni (vagina), so the upper part of it can be struck with the lingam (penis).
- **Churning:** Man holds his lingam with his hand and turns it around in his partner's yoni
- **Rubbing:** Similar as piercing, but involving the lower part of the yoni
- **Giving a Blow:** Man removes his lingam away from the yoni, and then brings it back to plunge deeply into the yoni with some force
- **Blow of a Boar:** Just one part of the yoni is rubbed by the lingam
- **Pressing:** The lingam is inserted into the yoni and pressed deep inside
- **Sporting of a Sparrow:** The lingam is inserted into the yoni and then moved up and down quickly without being withdrawn
- **Blow of a Bull:** The lingam rubs both sides of the yoni

Premature Ejaculation

Premature ejaculation is a problem that affects a lot of men. Most studies estimate that between 25 percent and 40 percent will face problems related to premature ejaculation at some point in their lives. This is by far the most common sexual problem, especially in men under forty years of age.

It can be tricky to define premature ejaculation with specific numbers, because the parameters vary from one man to another. For example, if a man (and his partner) is usually satisfied after ten minutes of sexual activity, then it is not really a problem if he tends to ejaculate shortly after that point. On the other hand, other men may consider it a problem if they ejaculate any sooner than the twenty-minute mark, or later. The bottom line: Premature ejaculation is generally used to refer to an occurrence where the man ejaculates way before he wants to, and before he wished to climax or conclude the sexual activity.

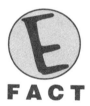

FACT

When trying to get to the root of a premature ejaculation problem, it is important to recognize whether this is a long-term chronic condition or something relatively new. If the man has always had this problem, this could signal a medical cause. If it just started recently, a psychological cause—or a new medical condition—could be to blame.

Causes of Premature Ejaculation

Premature ejaculation can be caused by a number of factors, both physical and psychological. In the majority of cases—especially where the man previously enjoyed a "normal" sex life and suddenly started having problems—a psychological cause is to blame. This may include severe "performance anxiety," depression, or stress. Occasionally a medical condition, such as a problem in the urinary tract, may be a factor.

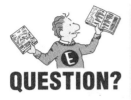

Is climaxing too quickly a sign of a medical problem?
Almost every man has an occasional experience where he climaxes too quickly, and this is nothing to be concerned with if it only happens once in a while. However, if it happens during a significant percentage of the man's sexual encounters, most experts would consider this a problem that needs to be addressed.

Effects of Premature Ejaculation

Technically, a man may be the only one who actually experiences premature ejaculation, but it can greatly affect his female partner, as well. She may be left frustrated and unsatisfied if the lovemaking session ends too quickly, before she has a chance to get "warmed up" or have an orgasm. Meanwhile, the man will have many negative emotions as well, including shame, frustration, anger, and embarrassment. Over time, this can end up causing a lot of stress and tension in the relationship. At the very least, the couple will find themselves less likely to even attempt to have sex, and pretty soon they may cease any sexual activity at all.

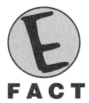

FACT

Mastering ejaculation control and multiple orgasm techniques can come in handy for any man, but can be especially beneficial for men who experience problems with premature ejaculation.

Treatment

The first step in treating a premature ejaculation problem is discussing it with your doctor. Do not be embarrassed—your doctor has almost surely heard about this from lots of patients before. Your doctor will want to get all the details on your general medical history, as well as your sexual history—particularly your sexual encounters coinciding with the start of this problem.

If a medical problem is suspected (which is relatively uncommon with regard to premature ejaculation), your doctor will probably refer you to a urologist or other specialist. More likely, though, your doctor will suspect a psychological culprit is to blame and will recommend that you consult a therapist or psychologist.

Most men find that a combination of therapy and sexual training techniques (which emphasize ejaculation delay and control) can be very effective in reducing or eliminating the problem. The good news? For the majority of men, this is a temporary problem that can be treated and/or cured, and a fulfilling sex life can soon be enjoyed again.

Erectile Dysfunction

Erectile dysfunction—often referred to as *impotence*—is a condition in which a man is unable to get or maintain a full erection. This condition is similar to premature ejaculation in that it can negatively affect both the man and his partner, and can put considerable strain on the relationship.

Erectile dysfunction can often be upsetting to the woman, who may fear that her partner is not excited because he does not find her sexy or attractive enough. The man, meanwhile, worries that he is somehow less of a man and will feel ashamed that he is unable to satisfy his partner.

Erectile dysfunction can also have an added complication, in that it can make it difficult or even impossible for the couple to conceive, which can be emotionally traumatic if the couple is trying to have a baby.

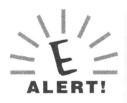

ALERT!

According to the National Institutes of Health, anywhere from 15 to 30 million men in the United States suffer from erectile dysfunction. According to the National Ambulatory Medical Care Survey, for every 1,000 men in the United States, 7.7 physician office visits were made for ED in 1985. By 1999, that rate had nearly tripled to 22.3.

Causes of Erectile Dysfunction

In trying to determine the possible cause of erectile dysfunction, the first factor a doctor will consider is the man's age. In older men, this problem is most likely brought on by a physical condition. Diseases—such as diabetes, kidney disease, chronic alcoholism, multiple sclerosis, atherosclerosis, vascular disease, and neurological disease—account for about 70 percent of ED cases, according to the National Institutes of Health. Diabetes is a huge risk factor; the NIH says between 35 and 50 percent of men with diabetes experience erectile dysfunction.

Smoking, obesity, and a sedentary lifestyle are also believed to increase a man's risk for erectile dysfunction. In addition, many common prescription medications—including antidepressants, diuretics, and drugs used to treat prostate cancer, high blood pressure, and Parkinson's disease—can have a side effect of erectile problems (as well as decreasing sex drive).

However, up to 20 percent of all cases of erectile dysfunction are believed to be linked to a psychological cause—including depression, performance anxiety, stress, and low self-esteem. If the man previously enjoyed a good sex life and only recently started to have erectile problems—especially if he is with a new partner, or he and his partner have been experiencing any problems in their relationship recently—this can point to emotional factors as a probable culprit.

Treatment

The good news is that erectile dysfunction is treatable in most men. Even better, scientific advancements have paved the way for several new drugs that are very successful in treating this condition. Usually a doctor will begin by pinpointing (and treating, wherever possible) any related medical conditions that could be causing the problem. He may also be able to adjust the patient's medications to alleviate side effects that include erectile dysfunction.

Frequently, the doctor will prescribe a prescription medication such as Viagra, Levitra, or Cialis, all of which have been successful in helping many men enjoy a thriving sex life again. If your doctor prescribes one of these medications for your man, you should make an effort to ensure he does not feel this is a sign of lessened manhood. Stress that this is nothing to be embarrassed about. (If it were, would all those pro athletes and high-profile figures willingly appear in ads for these products?)

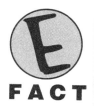

FACT

Just a few short years ago, most people had never heard of Viagra. Today, it has become a cultural phenomenon, with actors and high-profile men like Hugh Hefner raving about the magical powers of "the little blue pill." The makers of Viagra claim it can work in as little as fourteen minutes and helps up to 80 percent of men who take it.

As with premature ejaculation, if a psychological cause is suspected, therapy and counseling can make a big difference. Often, there is some underlying emotional or psychological problem. A therapist may also discover that the man has some sort of issue with his partner—some kind of negative feelings, which he may not even be consciously aware of—that is the hidden cause of the problem.

Increasing Libido

Although sagging libido is stereotypically viewed as a female problem, men can suffer from a slow sex drive as well. It is commonly believed that men reach their sexual peak in their teens or twenties, which means it would not be surprising if their libido took a slow but steady decline after that point.

Indeed, a man's testosterone levels (which are connected to his sex drive) do slowly decline starting at around age thirty.

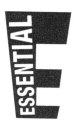

Many people believe that certain foods can help boost a man's libido. For example, the chemicals in celery are rumored to help spark a man's sex drive. Almonds and avocados are also said to have libido-boosting qualities. These foods are all pretty tasty, so why not give it a try and see what happens?

While there are lots of folk remedies—as well as a ton of trendy new products—that claim to boost a man's libido, most of these really don't work. However, there are a few natural ingredients that are considered to be helpful in this area—including ginseng, zinc, and vitamins A, C, and E. It is also a good idea to consult with your doctor to rule out any medical conditions that may be affecting your sex drive.

Enhancing Male Pleasure

For most men, sex (of any duration or variety) is so exciting and pleasurable that he is almost sure to have at least a somewhat enjoyable time even without any extra effort on your part. However, if your man makes an effort to please you, it is important for you to make his pleasure a priority as well. It is imperative to maintain this balance in the relationship, so there is a constant circle of give and take, as opposed to one partner always getting all of the pleasure.

Show Some Enthusiasm

One of the best things you can do to make sure your man has a good time? Show him that *you* are having a good time. Broadcast your pleasure loud and clear, in no uncertain terms. It is a huge turn-on for a man to watch his woman get aroused—especially if he knows he has played a part in it. One of men's biggest turnoffs is a woman who is too quiet or reserved in bed. Men are often a bit imperceptive when it comes to subtle clues, so he may not realize how much you are enjoying yourself unless you make it very clear.

You should leave no doubt in his mind that you are having a great time. He will become aroused just seeing how excited you are. Be sure to stress that you are excited because of *him*. It will be a huge boost to his ego knowing that he can get you so excited.

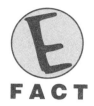

There are numerous sexual aids and toys—including penis rings—designed especially for a man's pleasure. You might consider picking up a few of these special treats without his knowledge. Save them for a special night, and then watch his excitement as he sees the surprises you have in store for him.

Focus on Him

While balance is important in achieving sexual harmony, it is perfectly okay to sometimes make it "his night." (Just be sure to even things out by also designating an equal number of "her night" occasions.) Arrange a special sacred area in which you will worship him. Announce that this night is all about focusing on his pleasure. Allow him to dictate the activities you engage in, and lavish him with even more attention and affection than usual. Treat him to a long session of fellatio, or whatever other activity he likes best. Throughout the evening, be sure to remind him repeatedly how sexy you think he is.

Chapter 21

Tantra Workshops and Classes

Hopefully this book will prove informative and helpful to you, but sometimes there is just no substitute for the in-person training and guidance you can get from attending a workshop or lecture. Some people simply learn and retain information better when it is being presented and demonstrated right in front of them. Fortunately, there are plenty of opportunities to learn about Tantra in person, as classes and events are held at lots of locations all across the country.

Why Take a Workshop?

While this book aims to be as complete and thorough as possible, some people simply learn and retain information better when it is presented verbally and visually through an in-person presentation. If you are one of those people, you will probably absorb a lot of additional material by attending a workshop or class. In addition, workshops and classes offer more specific material and individualized one-on-one attention that a book cannot provide. Not to mention, you will be following Tantric tradition. Remember, historically, Tantra was passed along through teachings imparted personally from a guru to his student.

Who You Are and What You Need

Before you start looking at your various options and figuring out which type of class might interest you, it is important to take stock of where you are in your Tantric journey, and in life in general.

Total Novice

Totally new to the teachings of Tantra? Don't be shy! You will be welcome at many workshops (obviously, steer clear of those designed specifically for people who are experienced and well-versed in Tantra). You might want to do some research beforehand, though (and reading this book is a good start) to get a basic overview of the topic and make sure it is something that interests you.

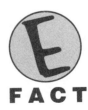

FACT

Most Tantric teachers and centers offer trial workshops or introductory classes. Some even allow you to buy videos or DVDs of past events. If possible, take advantage of these opportunities. It will give you a chance to observe the experience and see if it's a good fit for you before you fully commit.

As a novice, you might want to slowly ease into your educational program. When you first begin, it is probably best to look for a workshop where the demonstrations are not overly explicit or hands-on, unless you feel very comfortable with that sort of approach.

You need to decide whether to look for group instruction or one-on-one teaching. That is simply a matter of personal preference. Some new students fear they will be intimidated by the individual attention of a teacher before they are ready (although this fear usually proves unfounded) and would prefer to be able to "blend in" as part of a crowd. Others may want the personal attention of a teacher who is focused solely on them and can answer their specific questions, tailoring the material and the approach to the specific student.

The Shy/Reclusive Type

Perhaps you are the type of person who tends to be shy or uncomfortable in crowds (especially when potentially embarrassing personal topics such as sex are being discussed). Or maybe you are simply more of a homebody, or someone whose schedule and/or family situation does not allow a lot of free time to attend events in-person. Whatever your situation, you are in luck. There are many Tantra workshops and classes these days that take place online or via long-distance instruction. Obviously, you won't get the benefits of seeing a demonstration right before your very eyes, but you can still get many benefits from this type of instruction.

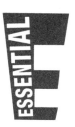

Some women feel more comfortable attending a Tantra workshop or class geared especially for female students. If you are female and nervous about going to a Tantra class, look for a "women only" event and enlist a few friends to go with you. Bonus: They will probably thank you for inviting them to this fun and enlightening event!

The Single Person

Not currently in a romantic relationship? No problem. You do not need to wait until you are "attached" to study Tantra. Single people are welcome in many classes and workshops. And in many ways, this may be the perfect time for you to pursue this new endeavor. You can focus all of your energy on your own spiritual and personal growth without worrying about neglecting a partner's needs. Plus, you will have a chance to reach an improved state of spiritual happiness before embarking on a new relationship. And when that perfect match does come along, you will be totally open and ready to share all of your Tantric wisdom.

In some ways, you may be at an advantage, in fact. This way, when you do find a "special someone," you will be able to introduce her or him to Tantric thinking right off the bat (assuming your new partner is not already familiar with Tantra). That is much easier than introducing new things to an in-progress relationship, where you need to teach an old dog new tricks.

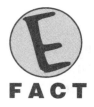

FACT

Here's a little secret: For single people, Tantra events can actually be a great place to meet new people, including perhaps a new partner. Some workshops devoted specifically to singles even incorporate a "meet-and-greet" type of gathering for just this purpose. Bonus: You know anyone you meet has a strong interest in Tantra. You already have something in common!

Many single people who do not want to attend Tantra events alone (or want to benefit from workshops geared toward couples) recruit a "learning buddy" to share the experience with them. This is a person who is not your partner romantically, but is someone you feel close to and comfortable with, and someone who shares your desire to learn this new philosophy.

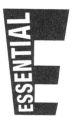

If you go to a Tantra workshop alone, there is a good chance the teachers will pair you up with another single attendee of the opposite sex to act as your study partner. If you would be uncomfortable with this, be sure to ask upfront about the policy for single participants.

Couples (Where Both Parties Are Interested)

If you are in a relationship, it is ideal if you both pursue this interest in Tantra together. Not only is it a great bonding experience that is almost guaranteed to strengthen your relationship, but you can also learn new things that you can then practice as a mutual activity. A lot of Tantra workshops are geared toward couples, and the majority of attendees later call this a wonderfully positive, fulfilling experience—something they are glad they shared with their partner.

Couples (With One Party Interested)

Even if your partner does not totally share your enthusiasm for Tantra at this time, do not be discouraged. It is perfectly okay to seek Tantric enlightenment all on your own. And here's a little secret: When one partner begins exploring the world of Tantra and then goes home and shares this newfound knowledge (and sensual techniques) with her partner, she often finds her partner to be a lot more receptive and interested in the whole concept.

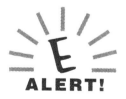

While most couples find the pursuit of Tantric teachings to be a profoundly strong bonding experience (even if one partner was not initially gung-ho about the idea), it can sometimes work in the opposite way. If your partner is extremely opposed to the idea, he may grow increasingly resentful of your new attitude and the personal changes in your spiritual beliefs.

The Tantra Veteran

Even if you are an experienced old pro when it comes to Tantra, you can still benefit from taking one or more Tantric workshop or class as a refresher course. Each instructor (or group of instructors) approaches the material with his or her own personal style and personality. And every workshop tends to be a bit different (even when presented by the same teacher), so it seems like you never walk away without learning something new. Not to mention, there's the opportunity to mingle and connect with other Tantric followers. And this is something that is always worth the price of any workshop admission.

Finding Classes or Workshops

So you have evaluated your situation and thought about what you want or need in a class. Now, how do you go about finding one? Fortunately, that part is pretty easy. Tantra workshops and classes are held all across the country, especially in larger cities. They are often held at Tantra centers or at universities or other facilities.

A simple online search for terms like "Tantra workshop" or "Tantric teacher" will yield lots of results. Enter your city (or the name of a major city near your location) to filter the results even further.

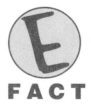

FACT

Some Tantra organizations are adding fun social elements to their educational events. For example, School of Tantra sponsors Club Tantra, where a Tantra class is followed by an intimate party for singles. If you are looking to make new friends (or find someone who wants to be more than friends), this might be a great opportunity for you.

You can also check the major Tantra Web sites such as Tantra.com. Most of them have a "Find a Teacher" link or section. Online Tantra clubs, discussion groups, or message boards are also a good way to find out about local Tantra events.

Even general online message boards such as Craigslist.org will often features news and information about Tantra events. Just use caution when searching for events through message boards not connected with a well-known reputable Tantra company. It is not unusual for people with less-than-honorable intentions to post "Tantra" ads on Craigslist.org, which are really just thinly disguised attempts at arranging a group sex get-together.

Interviewing a Potential Teacher

The good news? There are a lot of people out there offering Tantra workshops, classes, and one-on-one instruction. The bad news? Not all of these people are qualified to teach this topic. Some "instructors" may barely know anything about the topic, while others may be downright rip-off artists. Before you waste your money and time on a worthless workshop, you should do your homework and find out as much as you can about the class and the person who will be teaching it.

Here is another reason it is important to interview a potential teacher: You need to make sure his particular style of Tantra meshes well with the variety of Tantra that you wish to learn. As you have learned in this book, there are lots of different interpretations of Tantra, each with its own individual techniques and approaches. Not surprisingly, every teacher has her own unique interpretation of Tantra and her own way of teaching it. Some instructors focus solely on the traditional Hindu and Buddhist teachings, while others take a more modern approach and also include Neo-Tantra and Western attitudes. And there are instructors who also incorporate extra topics like yoga, dance, meditation, etc., into their material. This does not mean one particular teacher's approach is any better or worse than another's. But if you have a specific Tantric approach in mind, you need to find a teacher who is of like mind. Otherwise, you will be wasting both of your time.

Ask about Experience Level

One of the main things you will want to know about a prospective Tantra teacher is how much experience she has with Tantra, both as a teacher and a practitioner. A few Tantra instructors actually have medical degrees or are licensed therapists and psychologists. At the other end of the spectrum, there are "instructors" who have simply taken a few correspondence courses. And it's not just the length of the experience that matters. You also will want to know about the type of training the teacher had, the specific Tantric philosophies he studied, and the gurus he studied under. The good news is, you can often learn much of this information simply by visiting the teacher's Web site. It may also be included in the instructor's brochures or other materials. In addition, you can ask for references of other students or clients who have used the instructor's services.

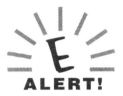

ALERT!

While Tantra workshops can help strength relationships and bring lovers closer together, they are not designed for major "relationship repair." Unless your instructor is a licensed therapist, she is not qualified to analyze or treat serious relationship problems. If you need this kind of help, seek out a professional counselor before you even consider going to a Tantra event.

Tantra Teaching Certifications

When evaluating a teacher, it can be helpful for you to know how a person goes about getting certified and/or qualified to teach Tantra. Unfortunately, there is really no official sanctioning body when it comes to overseeing Tantra teachers, but several of the larger Tantra centers and groups do have their own individual training/certification programs. For example, the Source School of Tantra (founded by Charles Muir three decades ago; it's one of the oldest such schools in the United States) trains and certifies instructors who then present their courses. The School of Tantra is another organization that trains and oversees Tantra instructors.

Do Your Research

Even if you get a good feeling (and good answers) from your prospective teacher, you may still feel the need for a bit more reassurance that this is right for you. Fortunately, it is easier than ever to do research on Tantra workshops—and just about everything else—these days. Most Tantra centers or instructors have their own Web sites where you can find lots of helpful information (often there is lots of information on Tantra in general, which may also prove very informative).

By doing an online search of the specific event and/or instructor, you can often find lots of background information and possibly even read reviews written by students who have studied with the instructor or taken the class previously. Even better, by browsing though online Tantra message boards or discussion groups, you may be able to "meet" and correspond personally with people who can provide firsthand information about the workshop.

How Hands-On Is It?

One of the most important things to consider when evaluating a Tantra program is the level of hands-on instruction that is involved. This can be a sensitive area, as some people (especially those new to the whole Tantric way of thinking) can be skittish about graphic demonstrations and/or those involving a lot of hands-on techniques.

With regard to this aspect, Tantra workshops can vary widely from one end of the spectrum to the other. Some workshops are lecture oriented, with minimal audience participation and no hands-on techniques involved. On the other hand, many workshops involve segments where you actually put the explained techniques into practice, either alone, with your partner, or with an instructor.

So as not to have any unpleasant or uncomfortable surprises, make sure you are clear beforehand about exactly what is involved.

You will be relieved to know, though, that Tantra teachers are generally very good at handling this situation. They are very respectful of people's fears and sensitivities, and will usually be very conscientious about respecting your boundaries, ensuring you are completely comfortable with any techniques.

Maximum Benefit Before and After the Workshop

Once you have found the perfect workshop for you, there are things you can do to help ensure you get the maximum benefits possible from the experience.

Before You Go

Before the workshop, preparation is the most important thing you can do. Obviously, some basic research on the general topic of Tantra is essential, but presumably you have already done that. At this point, you should also research the teacher and workshop as much as possible to familiarize yourself with both, which will make you feel more comfortable at the event.

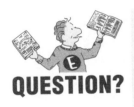

QUESTION?

Do attendees have to dress a certain way for a class?
For some Tantra classes, attendees must wear certain types or styles of clothing. This is especially common with courses involving a lot of hands-on activities, where it is usually advised to wear loose, comfortable clothes. Even if no dress code is specified, it is best to wear something that will allow you to relax and feel comfortable.

You should also ask about any special items you need to bring with you. Some interactive workshops require props such as a scarf, blindfold, or other items. It might also be a good idea to bring along a notebook so you can jot down any important information or tips. If the session features a lot of demonstrations, you might even want to ask if it would be okay for you to bring a camera. (This would allow you to show the highlights to your partner afterward, if he or she could not attend the event with you.)

After the Event

Following the Tantra event, you should take some time to review and contemplate all of the materials and information you have been given. There can often be a lot to digest, especially if you are a Tantra novice, so give yourself ample opportunity to go through the material step-by-step so you do not feel overwhelmed.

Cultivate Your Contacts

One of the best parts about attending a Tantra event is meeting lots of great people who share your interest in spiritual and sensual topics. Ideally, you met a few new friends with whom you might want to keep in touch. Perhaps they will even want to join you in attending your next Tantra event. This is a great way to build an exciting new social network of like-minded friends.

And don't forget the teacher—if you enjoyed the class, send a note or e-mail letting the instructor know. He will appreciate your feedback.

Continue Your Education

When it comes to spiritual enlightenment, you can never have too much education. So, now that you have gotten your first (or most recent) Tantra event under your belt, keep your eye open for other opportunities.

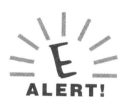

ALERT!

Not impressed with your first Tantra class? Don't be discouraged. This type of experience is a matter of personal taste, and perhaps this particular instructor or class did not suit your style. Look for other events with a different approach. Most likely, within the first few tries, you will find an event that is just what you're looking for.

Things to Keep in Mind

You will get the most out of your Tantra learning experience if you are fully prepared and know what to expect. So here are a few more pieces of advice.

Don't Be Afraid to State Your Preferences

Not every teacher is a good fit for every student. If there is a certain instructor or type of instructor you prefer (for example, if you feel more comfortable with a teacher of the same gender as you), you should feel free to speak up. A good Tantra instructor will not mind or be offended at all. Most likely, she has heard the same questions or requests many times in the past. Tantra teachers are aware that this is a very personal spiritual experience, one in which a good personal connection and rapport with the instructor is essential. The staff should try to do whatever they can to make you feel most at ease. So, if you prefer to have a specific instructor, just say so. Obviously, this mainly applies to Tantra centers with a group of staff members, or events where more than one instructor will be on hand.

Costs and Time Commitments Vary Widely

Like most people, you probably have limited time as well as a tight budget. Neither should be an obstacle in your quest for Tantric knowledge. When it comes to Tantra instruction, you can invest as much or as little time and money as you wish. Short classes—especially the lecture variety that are often presented at local colleges—tend to be pretty cheap. Also, events where there is a large group of attendees are generally more affordable on a per-person basis. As a general rule, the smaller the group, the higher the cost will be for each attendee. Obviously, individual one-on-one instruction can be somewhat pricier.

Likewise, the time commitment can really vary. You can attend a single one-hour lecture, or a week-long Tantra excursion. There are programs where you attend instruction for six or more hours per day, for several days in a row. Obviously, this type of program is not for everyone. You need to be really committed and have a chunk of available time (not to mention money—this type of program can cost $2,000 or more).

Make It a Vacation

If you have some available time, and a little bit of money to spend, consider taking a Tantra vacation. This is where your trip does double-duty: It is a getaway from the daily stresses of everyday life, but is also a great way to get some in-depth Tantra training. If you are in a committed relationship, bring your partner. This will make for a wonderful romantic getaway, and you can study Tantric techniques together. Services like Intimacy Retreats (see their information in the Resources section of this book) specialize in

Tantra getaway vacations in exotic locations like Hawaii. Female readers will be interested to know that there are also some women-only retreats in exotic locations. This would be a great "girls-only getaway" for you and a group of friends. And, who knows, you just might meet a sexy Hawaiian hunk while strolling along the beach in between seminars.

Chapter 22

Tantra for Special Categories of People

Tantra does not discriminate. All human beings, from all walks of life, are seen as equally valuable and worthy of love and respect. The Tantra community prides itself on being welcoming and accepting of all people, regardless of their background, lifestyle, age, or other factors. It is truly one big melting pot of sacred love. There are some groups of people, though, who may be especially in need of the wonderful things Tantra can offer.

Who Is Tantra For?

Tantra is for anyone with a sincere desire to learn and improve her or his life through Tantric practices. Tantra is studied by a vastly diverse group of people. Everyone is welcome, and nobody should feel out of place or unwanted. People of all shapes, sizes, and varieties can reap countless benefits from Tantric teachings. However, there are specific groups of people for whom Tantra can offer particular advantages.

Different Age Groups

You might say that Tantra does not recognize age. Remember, Tantrics believe we are all spiritual, worldly beings, so the chronological age of our earthly bodies is almost irrelevant. However, for many people, age is an issue. And there are certain age categories that seem to need something special from Tantra.

College Students

For college students (and people in their twenties in general), romance can be confusing. And spirituality can be even tougher. This is a period of life where it is all about finding yourself, discovering your place in this world. Young people are constantly seeking the meaning of life, and looking for a higher meaning. The younger generation of today is also keenly interested in ancient philosophies and belief systems. Tantra can satisfy their thirst for the ancient secrets of life.

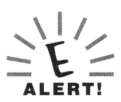

ALERT!

Disappointed to find that there are no Tantra events near your college or on your campus? Take action! Ask around, and see how you could go about starting a Tantra club or bringing in a Tantric teacher to speak or present a workshop. You will be a hero to all the people who will soon discover the magic of Tantra.

From a sexual standpoint, this can be a great age to study Tantra. Young people are exploring their sexuality but have not yet fully developed their sexual routines. So they do not have as many "bad bedroom habits" to break as someone would at an older age. By mastering Tantric techniques at this age, they will incorporate the techniques into their regular romantic routines, and quickly adapt to them so well that Tantric ways become automatic. College-aged women today, being of an independent and empowered nature, will really like the Tantric emphasis on female power.

In addition, today's college students of both genders tend to be very conscious of the world around them. Tantra's emphasis on balance with nature and respect for the environment and the world around you fits nicely with the social causes and interests favored by many young people.

Young Parents

Young parents do not have it easy today. They are taking care of several young kids, running a household, and most likely juggling careers, all of which leaves them feeling overwhelmed and overworked, yet underappreciated. For these busy parents, romance is a distant memory—which is especially sad, considering many of them have only been together a few years. Busy parents like these often neglect their own relationship, letting their personal life suffer in order to put their children and careers first.

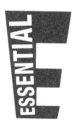

New parents often have trouble maintaining their social life, especially if they "outgrew" their previous circle of friends after having a child. Parents who want to meet new friends (or reconnect with old ones) and also explore Tantra can combine the two by hosting a fun at-home adult party through a company like Passion Parties. It's a fun get-together (think a sexier version of a Tupperware party).

Tantra can be a godsend to this group. Tantra will teach them the importance of recapturing the romance in their relationship. They can learn how to once again feel like the young lovers that they still are. They will also learn how taking care of their own needs will actually make them better parents, because they will feel happier and more fulfilled. And of course the stress-relieving Tantra techniques of meditation and yoga can really come in handy for this group.

Baby Boomers

The baby boomers are a population segment that is, well, booming. Baby boomers are what some might not-so-gently refer to as middle aged. But baby boomers do not think of themselves that way. They consider themselves vibrant, energetic, fun-loving people who enjoy life.

However, a lot of baby boomers do have some specific circumstances in their life that can prove to be challenging. Many are divorced and navigating the dating scene for the first time in years, possibly since their college days. Others may have lost a spouse, and find themselves a widow or widower way earlier than they ever expected.

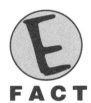

FACT

A survey of 2,000 married baby boomers conducted by Harris International found that 84 percent of them considered physical intimacy as being "important or very important." Unfortunately, only half of the respondents were satisfied with the level of physical intimacy in their relationship.

These people, to put it bluntly, have probably fallen into a rut. There is a good chance they have been (or had been) with the same partner for many years. Most likely, they fell into a comfortable—maybe even boring—routine in the bedroom. For people of this generation (especially women) sex is not a topic they talked about a lot as young people. Their sexual insight may still be fairly limited, especially if they and their partner were both relatively inexperienced when they began their relationship all those years ago.

This group may find Tantra to be a real eye-opener. The sexual freedom and emphasis on passion may be liberating in a powerful way. They may find themselves enjoying pleasure like they never imagined.

For men of this generation, they may have been brought up with outdated, old-fashioned ideas about sex. Most likely, they never learned to focus on a woman's pleasure before worrying about their own. They may be eager to learn new tricks for satisfying their female partner. As for the women, they will be thrilled at this new attitude in their partner. They will also welcome the opportunity to learn a few new tricks of their own. While they may have been more timid and sexually inhibited in the past, they can now show off a more liberated, sexually adventurous side of themselves.

Since people at this stage often no longer have young children at home, this can be the perfect time to focus on their own needs and desires, and concentrate on their relationships and happiness.

Different Lifestyles

From a Tantric viewpoint, we all have one common lifestyle: sensual and spiritual. We each put those aspects into action in different ways, through the lifestyle path we choose. Tantra—especially Neo-Tantra—embraces all lifestyle options, believing one should follow whatever path is right for his or her soul.

Gay and Bisexual

It is true that, according to many gurus, traditional Tantra was not exactly supportive and encouraging where homosexuality was involved. Ancient texts reportedly warned of the dangers of male homosexuality (also known as reverse kundalini) and stressed the negative physical and psychological effects of this type of sex.

However, views have evolved on that issue. Modern Tantra does not view homosexuality or bisexuality as anything to be scorned, ridiculed, or viewed as foreign. Although Tantric texts stress the importance of male and female union, this does not need to be interpreted literally. It can also be taken to mean the union of male and female spirits, both of which live inside each of us. At most Tantra events, there are quite a few gay and bisexual participants and attendees. There are even workshops and retreats specifically geared toward those in same-sex relationships.

Couples Who Practice Polyamory

Earlier in this book, the practice of polyamory was discussed in great detail. People who practice a polyamorous lifestyle believe in loving many, which often translates into sexual union with a number of different partners. This is similar to what many people not familiar with polyamory might also call "swinging," although the two lifestyles have very different philosophies. Because this lifestyle is unconventional, it is often seen as strange or perverted, and the people who practice it may find themselves the target of ridicule, scorn, or discrimination. As a result, they are often forced to be very discreet, keeping their lifestyle a secret from the world around them.

But for polyamorous people, Tantra can be a safe haven. There are numerous members of the Tantric community who practice polyamory as a lifestyle, so this is not viewed as something weird or unusual. People who practice polyamory will find themselves welcome. In fact, there are many events, Web sites, and clubs devoted exclusively to Tantra for polyamorous people.

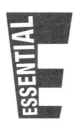

To learn more about polyamory and the people who practice it, visit the Web site of the Polyamory Society at ✐*www.polyamorysociety.org*. You can learn all about legal and advocacy issues relating to polyamory, locate support groups and events, and get tips on how to explain your polyamorous lifestyle (or how to handle it when a loved one announces his or hers).

Physical Characteristics

We live in a world where image and physical appearance are everything. Or at least, that is how it often seems. It can often seem like the beautiful people—those who fit a certain mold—have all of the fun, while those who are self-conscious about their looks get left in the shadows. Fortunately, Tantra does not adhere to this way of thinking. Tantra welcomes everyone, without giving appearance a single thought.

Body Issues

Many people have issues with their bodies. This is especially true for women, but a surprising number of men are very self-conscious about their bodies, too. Weight-related issues are probably the most common, but people can also be self-conscious about being too short or tall, too pale or dark, or have any number of other issues relating to their physical appearance.

The singles scene is stressful enough for anyone, but when you add serious body issues to the mix, dating can be a disaster. It can be scary just to mingle with people, let alone actually removing your clothes in front of someone.

For people with body concerns, Tantra can be an answer to their prayers. Tantra stresses the importance of the human body—any human body, whatever its shape or form. All human bodies are seen as beautiful and worthy of worship. There is no image of "perfect" beauty. Tantra does not promote a cookie-cutter ideal of physical appearance. A woman is a goddess, regardless of the shape of her physical form. The same thing is true for a man. If you glance through books on Tantra that feature old Tantra drawings and illustrations, you will see people of all physical types depicted, and all of them are seen as sexy and desirable.

Tantra's goal is to achieve a spiritual union, a cosmic harmony. At that level of consciousness, physical appearance is a nonissue. All that is important is the soul and spirit. You are a divine being who transcends any physical characteristics.

By following Tantric philosophies, you can have a fulfilling sex life, and enjoy lots of romance, regardless of your body type. And by embracing your inner god or goddess, you will learn to love yourself exactly as you are—a beautiful godlike human being.

Racial and Ethnic Diversity

Just as Tantra does not differentiate people according to dress size, the Tantra way of life also does not categorize people according to skin color or nationality. Human beings are not judged by the color of the body that their spirit happens to inhabit. It does not matter, from a Tantric acceptance standpoint, what your racial or ethnic profile is. You are worthy of love, honor, and respect.

Mismatched Couples

If you go to enough Tantra events, you will start to notice an unusual phenomenon. Many of the couples look, well, like they don't really fit together in the conventional sense. You will often spot people from different backgrounds, of different races, and from different age groups all paired together in happily committed relationships. It may catch you off guard, leaving you wondering if you have somehow stumbled onto a game of romantic musical chairs, where the people have all been scrambled from their "correct" partners.

This is actually a very common trend. Veteran Tantrics do not even bat an eyelash at this anymore, because they have grown so accustomed to it. This is a testament to Tantra's encouraging attitude toward diversity and acceptance. When you think about it, the mismatched couple trend is actually very fitting for Tantra. After all, this is a philosophy whose core principle is the union of two halves, the joining of opposite sides. Tantra is all about the balance of yin and yang, of the feminine and masculine joining in harmony. So, with that in mind, it seems to make perfect sense that people who are seemingly total opposites would fit together perfectly, complementing each other as no other partner would.

Indeed, as any Tantra teacher will tell you, this even happens at events where Tantra serves as a "matchmaker." At Tantra events for singles, it can be amusing to see people pair up. Often the least likely combinations of people will gravitate toward each other. And it is not unusual for these mismatched couples to have an instant spark and form a close bond.

People with Disabilities

For people with disabilities, dating is often a challenge—and sex can often seem downright impossible, if not physically then definitely psychologically. For people with disabilities, their physical limitations often leave them feeling powerless or less worthy than more able-bodied people.

Again, this is where Tantra—with its focus on the spiritual part of the person, not the physical—can be a lifesaver. Tantra values the human spirit, no matter what physical limitations its body may have. Also, Tantra's focus on sensual activities—not just the act of intercourse—can help people enjoy a sensual, romantic relationship, regardless of whatever physical limitations they may have. And with all of the countless sexual positions in the Tantric repertoire, there is surely at least one or two that almost anyone can enjoy—perhaps with a bit of creativity and determination.

Psychological and Emotional Issues

With its focus on spiritual strength, as well as physical well-being and the mind-body connection, Tantra can be a help to anyone with issues related to their psychological or emotional well-being. This is enhanced by the fact that Tantra stresses the importance of nurturing your soul and attending to your own emotional health.

Sexual Healing

A lot of people have had a sexual crisis or trauma in their lives. This may have led to sexual dysfunction or major inhibitions. In turn, that often leads to a very unfulfilling love life. In many cases, the person may abandon sex altogether. Fortunately, Tantra promotes sexual healing. It helps people overcome the sexual problems they may have experienced and brings a bright new light back to their lives. They will gradually heal their wounds and begin to see sex in a refreshingly positive way.

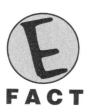

FACT

Tantra can be especially beneficial to people who have experienced emotional pain or trauma, or anyone who has been through a trying ordeal. The soothing, loving, and nurturing aspects of Tantra can provide a recovery process that can be a lifesaver to those who need emotional healing.

Past Abusive Relationships

For people who have been in abusive relationships in the past, embarking on a new romantic start can be a very scary prospect. Tantra can help because it encourages strength and power, which is especially important for female survivors of past abuse. For someone who has been belittled, abused, or mistreated, being in a relationship where they are treated as a goddess is a breath of fresh air and positive energy. It is a rebirth and a new beginning. They will slowly realize that—despite what their abuser led them to believe—they are worthy of love and affection, along with respect and kindness.

Appendix A

Glossary

Ajna
The chakra located on the forehead; also known as "the third eye." It correlates to intuition.

Amrita
Female ejaculatory fluid. Considered a desirable "life force" and known in Tantra as "nectar of a goddess." Based on a Sanskrit term meaning "elixir of immortality."

Anahata
Chakra located near the heart. Symbolizes love, joy, and happiness.

Asana
Yoga pose or posture, used to exercise the body and refresh the spirit.

Ayurveda
A system of medicine and healing that can be traced back to ancient India; a holistic spiritual approach.

Bandhas
Postures employed in yoga that constrict specific parts of the body.

Bliss
A state of ultimate happiness and contentment; often illustrated as a powerful light filling the body and soul.

Bon
Indigenous religion of Tibet.

Burton, Richard
British scholar, linguist, and explorer who translated the first English version of the Kama Sutra.

Chakra
Energy center. Based on the Sanskrit term meaning "circle" or "wheel." There are seven energy centers associated with the human body.

Chakra Puja
Also known as group worship, an ancient Tantric ritual involving up to eight couples. Literally translated to mean "circle worship."

Chang, Stephen Thomas
Author of *The Tao of Sexology*, he is credited with coining the term *million dollar point*.

Chi
A Chinese term for spiritual energy; sometimes used to refer to air or breath.

Consort
Spouse or sexual partner, usually connected to royalty or someone in an important position of power.

Deity
Divine being; god; being of significant power; someone thought to be holy or sacred.

Doshas
Unique combination of fundamental energies. There are three main doshas: vata (air and space), kapha (water and earth), and pitta (fire).

Ejacularion
The deliberate avoidance of ejaculation.

Enlightenment
State of ultimate consciousness and higher awareness.

Feng shui
Home building and decorating approach based on the idea of living in harmony with your environment and surroundings.

FSAD
Female sexual arousal disorder; a condition in which a woman experiences little or no desire for sex.

God/goddess
A religious deity; also, refers to all men and women, who are all deserving of reverence and respect.

Great rite
Wiccan ritual that involves the union (symbolic or physical) between two people.

Guru
Teacher or spiritual guide. Ancient gurus were viewed with the highest respect and believed to be supremely wise beings. Based on the Sanskrit term for "dispeller of ignorance."

Inner flute
Energy pathway through the body that follows the path of the chakras and is said to enable deep breathing.

Jiao
Type of ritual practiced in Taoism.

Jing
Sexual reproductive drive that Taoists believed should be harnessed and used for better health and happiness.

Jnana mudra
Fantasy partner, who is present only in the imaginer's mind; also a sacred Tantric hand gesture.

Kama Sutra
Very well-known ancient Hindu sex guide.

Kapala
Skull cup used as a bowl to contain food or liquids that will be offered in a symbolic sacrifice. Traditionally made from an actual skull, but in modern times a cup that simply resembles a skull has become acceptable.

Karma
The principle of universal cause and effect.

Karma mudra
Traditional Buddhist Tantra term for a sex partner.

Kegel, Arnold
California gynecologist and obstetrician credited with discovering Kegel exercises in the 1940s.

Kegel exercises
Exercises designed to strengthen the PC muscles in the pelvis region. Usually involves contracting and holding the muscles for brief intervals.

Karezza
The term for the Tantric technique of learning to control the orgasm response using various techniques including breathing routines and finger pressure. Sometimes also used to refer to sacred sex in general.

Kumari
Sanskrit term for a female virgin.

Kumari Puja
Tantric ritual involving the worship of a virgin girl.

Kundalini
Sexual energy or power; based on a Sanskrit work meaning "pool of energy." Often depicted in the form of a serpent.

Lingam
The penis, also known in Tantra as the "wand of light" or "magic wand."

Maithuna
Sanskrit term for union; often used to refer to sexual union.

Maithuna Sadhana
A Tantric sexual ritual, also known as "the secret rite," which involved proceeding through a lovemaking encounter in a deliberate, pre-established timeline and sequence of events.

Mala
A string of rotary beads, similar in appearance to those used by people of the Christian faith.

Mandala
A sacred circle, frequently embellished with jewels or precious metals; believed to hold secrets about life and death; used in conjunction with meditation.

Manipura
Chakra located in the abdomen. It is associated with feelings of control and anger.

Mantra
Chant or incantation, often used in meditation; it is believed the repetitive chanting helps one's mental focus.

Million dollar point
Specific spot in a man's perineum that ancient people believed could block the flow of seminal fluid.

Mudras
Ritual Tantric hand gestures designed to help focus the body's energy; often used in conjunction with meditation.

Muir, Charles
Self-proclaimed "grandfather of the modern Tantra movement in the United States." Creator of the "Tantra: The Art of Conscious Loving" format of Tantric instruction, based on a book he cowrote with his wife.

Muladhara
Chakra located in the genital region. This is the base chakra. It is often equated with life.

Neo-Tantra
Also known as westernized Tantra, a form of Tantra that focuses less on the ancient spiritual traditions and more on the sexual aspects.

Osho
Well-known and controversial twentieth-century Indian spiritual guide and teacher.

Padmasambhava
Highly revered figure in Buddhist history. Founder of the Tantric School of Buddhism.

Pancha Karma
Multistep process of cleansing the body and ridding it of toxins.

PC (pubococcygeal) muscles
Pelvic muscles (in both men and women), which can be strengthened through contracting exercises—called Kegel exercises—in order to provide enhanced sexual abilities, as well as better pelvic conditioning.

Phurpha
Sacred magic dagger often used in Tantric rituals, and believed to help defeat evil spirits.

Playing the flute
Tantric term for oral sex performed on a man.

Polishing the pearl
Tantric term for oral sex performed on a woman.

Pompoir
Ancient Chinese art in which a woman "milks" her partner's penis by tightly squeezing her PC muscles during sexual union.

Prana
Breath or energy; based on the Sanskrit term for "life force."

Puja
Hindu ritual of worship.

Reverse kundalini
A Tantric term used to refer to any sexual technique viewed as unnatural or against the norm.

Rite of the Five Essentials
A Tantric sexual ritual involving five essential elements: meat, fish, wine, grains, and sexual union. Also known as "the Tantric Eucharist" or "the Ritual of the Five M's."

Sacrament
Sacred item or activity, often used in rituals. Ancient Tantrics sometimes engaged in rituals involving five sacraments: meat, fish, wine, grains, and sexual union.

Sacred sex
Sexual encounters using Tantric approaches or techniques.

Sacred space
A special area dedicated to lovemaking and romantic connections with a partner.

Sahasrara
Chakra located at the top of the head, also known as the crown chakra. It represents a person who is god-like and also symbolizes one's connection to God.

Sanskrit
Believed to be one of the oldest human languages; the Hindu language in which most ancient religious texts are written.

Sexual union
Tantric term for intercourse.

Shakti
Hindu goddess; the creative life force; also feminine energy.

Shiva
Hindu god; the essential principle of pure consciousness. Also used to refer to a man who is viewed as embodying male energy and a powerful masculine force.

Siddha
Sanskrit term meaning someone who has attained a "grand master" type of status.

Siddhartha Gautama
Buddha from Nepal born during sixth century B.C. Tantra and other types of Buddhism trace their roots back to his teachings. His beliefs centered around the idea of the "middle path," which stressed balance and moderation.

Swadhisthana
Chakra located between the navel and groin. It is associated with the qualities of emotion and sexuality.

Tantra
Ancient system of philosophical beliefs based on the quest for supreme bliss. The term *Tantra* is Sanskrit for "weave" or "woven together." Tantra originated in ancient India and later spread to other areas including China, Tibet, and Nepal.

Tantric
A person who practices Tantra; also *Tantrika* or *Tantrica*.

Taoism
Ancient Chinese philosophy that views nature and spiritualism as two independent entities. The word *Tao* is Chinese for "the way."

Theravada
The traditional branch of Buddhism stresses strict discipline and self-denial and frowns upon the sexual rituals common in Tantric Buddhism.

Third eye
Tantric symbol of higher consciousness; also known as "the mind's eye."

Vajra
One of the primary Tantric symbols, the vajra is generally believed to be a combination of a scepter and some kind of weapon. It represents the quality of being strong and indestructible. Also used as another term for the penis.

Vajrayana
Tantric Buddhism, also known as Tibetan Buddhism.

Vastu
The ancient Indian science of design and architecture.

Vatsyayana
Ancient guru credited with creating the Kama Sutra.

Vedas
Large collection of sacred texts from ancient India.

Vishuddha
Chakra located at the base of the throat. Symbolizes communication and self-expression.

Yab yum
The most famous Tantric love position, in which the couple sits facing each other, their bodies entwined with the woman sitting in the man's lap.

Yang
Chinese term for the male half of a pair, or masculine characteristics. Also referred to as "the Force of Heaven."

Yantra
Geometric drawing representing beauty and seen as having sacred meaning because its pattern represents a deity; a symbol of divine power. Ancient people believed mystical yantras that could reveal secrets of the universe. Sexual positions are sometimes also referred to as yantras.

Yin
Chinese term meaning the feminine half of a pair; also referred to as "the Force of Earth."

Yoga
A discipline designed to connect the physical and spiritual systems, and encourage a stronger connection with the universe, promoting a higher state of consciousness; based on the Sanskrit term for "to join together."

Yogi
Someone who teaches yoga or is very proficient in yoga techniques.

Yoni
Sanskrit term for vagina.

Appendix B

Tantric Facts and Fallacies

Tantra is a subject surrounded by misinformation and misconceptions. Here are some facts and fallacies related to this ancient Indian system of beliefs.

Tantra is a new sexual trend.
False. Tantra has actually been around for thousands of years.

Tantra was created by Americans.
False. Tantra was a widespread practice in ancient India and Tibet. In fact, Americans were among the last people to discover Tantra.

Hindu Tantra places a greater emphasis on rituals than does the Buddhist version of Tantra.
True, at least for rituals involving sex.

People who practice Tantra engage in reckless behavior and unsafe sexual practices.
False. While there are always exceptions, most Tantrics are very careful about their health, take all the necessary precautions, and consider safe sex practices to be a top priority.

Tantra involves sorcery, witchcraft, and black magic.
False, for the most part. This was a common misconception among people of ancient times, leading to unfair prejudices against Tantrics. Some Tantric sects do involve such things—although not many.

Tantra stresses promiscuous behavior.
False. Tantra encourages people to pursue whatever sexual path they feel is true to their spirit. Tantrics include celibates, monogamous couples, couples who practice polyamory, and people of many other lifestyles.

Tantra is a religion, requiring followers to denounce other religions.
False. Tantra is a system of philosophical beliefs, not a religion. It is practiced by people of all different religious faiths. You do not need to

"renounce" your current church or religion in order to be accepted by the Tantric community.

Taoists believed a man should ejaculate as often as possible to prove his manhood.

False. Ejaculation was viewed as a waste of precious life forces, and was to be avoided whenever possible. In fact, many Taoists, especially in past centuries, practiced ejacularion (the deliberate avoidance of ejaculation).

The Kama Sutra is a Tantric sexual how-to guide.

False. Although the two are often closely linked, the Kama Sutra was primarily a guide for relationships between men and women, including sexual interaction. It does include some sexual techniques that can be used during Tantric lovemaking.

Tantra promotes strange rituals involving sex.

False—mostly. It is true that ancient Tantras often practiced rituals focusing on sexual unions, but this has largely become a thing of the past. Modern Tantrics, however, do practice sexual rituals of a positive nature, such as setting a romantic mood with sensual baths or erotic massage.

Tantra is only for young people.

False. People of all ages can enjoy (and benefit from) all that Tantra has to offer. An increasing number of baby boomers—and, yes, even senior citizens—are discovering the difference that Tantra can make in their lives and in their relationships.

Tantra is for people in the big cities.

False. People from all over the country (and, of course, all over the world) practice Tantra. No matter where you live, it is very likely that there are many Tantrikas nearby. If there are not any Tantra workshops or events close to you, that is not a problem—you can study Tantra online, and also participate in Web forums and online communities.

Tantra promotes good physical health.

True. Many of the practices encouraged by Tantra—including yoga, meditation, and deep breathing—can have major physical benefits. Since Tantrics often have a strong connection to nature, they also frequently practice healthy eating habits involving organic foods and vegetarianism.

Tantra events are open only to straight, married couples.

False. Tantra workshops are known for their welcoming attitude toward everyone. Generally, people from all lifestyles are welcome. There are also some events geared specifically toward certain demographics, such as gay men or polyamorous couples.

Appendix C

Resources

Web Sites

www.tantra.com—considered the ultimate online Tantric resource. Features advice, articles, interviews, discussion forums, and an online store offering many different sensual items.

www.tantraattahoe.com—site of Tantrics Somraj and Jeffre, who specialize in teaching Supreme Bliss Tantra. Find out about personal training and coaching services, order e-books, enroll in online courses, and browse their catalog of adult products.

www.robintaylor.net—site of sexologist and counselor Robin Taylor, who offers workshops and private Tantra coaching sessions.

www.sourcetantra.com—site of well-known Tantra teachers Charles and Caroline Muir. They specialize in workshops and retreats for couples—including a great weeklong vacation seminar in Hawaii. You can also register for a home study course or maybe even look into becoming a certified Tantra teacher yourself.

www.tantra-sex.com—site of veteran Tantra teachers and author Al Link and Pala Copeland. This comprehensive site includes articles, interviews, private workshops, e-books, CDs, books, and erotic products.

www.margotanand.com—site of Sky Dancing Tantra and Margot Anand, considered a modern Tantra pioneer.

www.ecstaticliving.com—site of the Institute for Ecstatic Living, as well as Steve and Lokita Carter, a California couple who teach Tantra workshops.

www.royalle.com—site of Candida Royalle and Femme Productions. Learn about this female pioneer in the sex industry, and order her women-friendly erotic movies or her Natural Contours adult toys.

www.adameve.com—site of the popular adult retailer Adam & Eve, where you can buy adult toys, erotic films, sensual clothing, and other products.

www.tantraworks.com—site of Nik Douglas, author of several books related to Tantra. Features a long list of resources and links.

www.tantratalk.com—online community and forum for the discussion of topics related to Tantra.

www.sexuality.org—information-packed resources for all topics related to sexuality. Includes dozens of documents on sexual subjects including Tantra, as well as oral sex, positions, and more.

www.lovemore.com—comprehensive site devoted to the polyamorous lifestyle. Features *Loving More Magazine*, plus information on polyamory conferences, books, and other resources.

www.passionparties.com—site of Passion Parties, a company that helps people host fun adult-themed parties in their home during which attendants can order adult merchandise.

www.devamusic.com—online source for music especially geared for massage, healing, meditation, and more. Features section for Tantra CDs.

www.aneros.com—site where you can order the Aneros Prostate Massager, which is designed to help men achieve powerful, dry, full-body orgasms in rapid succession.

www.loverocker.com—site where you can order furniture designed for sexual encounters.

www.loving-angles.com—site where you can order furniture that can easily be arranged in numerous different configurations, especially for various sexual positions.

www.wantedlist.com—service that allows you to rent adult movies by mail, keeping them as long as you like for a monthly fee.

Books

Anand, Margot. *The Art of Sexual Ecstasy.* (Tarcher/Penguin, 1989).

Anderson, Bruce. *Tantra for Gay Men.* (Alyson Books, 2002).

Beer, Robert. *The Encyclopedia of Tibetan Symbols and Motifs.* (Shambhala, 1999).

Brockway, Laurie Sue. *A Goddess Is a Girl's Best Friend: A Divine Guide to Finding Love, Success and Happiness.* (Perigee Books).

Brooks, Valerie. *Tantric Awakening: A Women's Initiation into the Path of Ecstasy.* (Destiny Books, 2001).

Camphausen, Rufus C. *The Encyclopedia of Sacred Sexuality.* (Inner Traditions, 1999).

Chopra, Deepak. *Deepak Chopra: Kama Sutra.* (Virgin Books, 2006).

Harding, Kat. *The Lesbian Kama Sutra.* (Thomas Dunne Books, 2006).

Hyatte, Christopher. *Secrets of Western Tantra*, 2nd ed. (New Falcon Publications, 1996).

Heumann, Suzie, and Susan Campbell. *The Everything Great Sex Book.* (Adams Media, 2004).

Iam, Mabel. *Sex and the Perfect Lover: Tao, Tantra and the Kama Sutra.* (Atria, 2006).

Inkeles, Gordon. *The New Sensual Massage.* (Arcata Arts, 1998).

Lacroix, Nitya. *The Art of Tantric Sex.* (DK Publishing, 1997).

Link, Al, and Pala Copeland. *Soul Sex: Tantra for Two.* (New Page Books, 2003); *Complete Idiot's Guide to Supercharged Kama Sutra.* (Alpha Books/Penguin, 2007); *Sensual Love Secrets for Couples: The Four Freedoms of Body, Heart, Mind and Soul.* (Llewellyn Worldwide, 2007); *Tantric Sex Step By Step: 28 Days to Ecstasy.* (Llewellyn Worldwide, 2007).

McKenzie, Eleanor. *The Kama Sutra Year: 52 Sensational Positions for Erotic Pleasure.* (Fair Winds Press, 2005).

Muir, Charles, and Caroline Muir. *Tantra: The Art of Conscious Loving.* (Mercury House, 1989).

Osho. *The Book of Secrets.* (St. Martin's Griffin, 1998).

Pokras, Somraj. Several e-books and courses available at *www.TantraAtTahoe.com.*

Ramsdale, David, and Cynthia W. Gentry. *Red Hot Tantra: Erotic Secrets of Red Tantra for Intimate, Soul-to-Soul Sex and Ecstatic, Enlightened Orgasms.* (Quiver, 2004).

Reynolds, Virginia. *A Lover's Guide to the Kama Sutra.* (Peter Pauper Press, 2002).

Richardson, Diana. *Tantric Orgasm for Women.* (Park Street Press, 2004).

Riley, Kerry. *Tantric Secrets for Men: What Every Woman Will Want Her Man to Know.* (Destiny Books, 2002).

Royalle, Candida. *How to Tell a Naked Man What to Do: Sex Advice from a Woman Who Knows.* (Simon & Schuster/Fireside, 2004).

Russell, Stephen. *The Tao of Sexual Massage: A Step-by-Step Guide to Exciting, Enduring, Loving Pleasure.* (Fireside, 2003).

Salnicki, Marcus. *The Art of Sensual Massage: Techniques to Awaken the Senses and Pleasure Your Partner.* (Sterling, 2004).

Sampson, Val. *Tantra Between the Sheets: The Easy and Fun Guide to Mind-Blowing Sex.* (Amorata Press, 2003).

Sarita, Ma Ananda, and Swami Anand Geho. *Tantric Love.* (Fireside, 2001).

Schulte, Christa. *Tantric Sex for Women: A Guide for Lesbian, Bi, Hetero and Solo Lovers.* (Hunter House, 2004).

Sonntag, Linda. *Bedside Kama Sutra Kit: Everything You Need for a Weekend of Absolute Passion.* (Fair Winds Press, 2003).

Stanway, Andrew. *Massage Secrets for Lovers: The Ultimate Guide to Intimate Arousal.* (Carroll & Graf, 2002).

Stubbs, Kenneth Ray. *The Essential Tantra: A Modern Guide to Sacred Sexuality.* (Tarcher/Penguin, 2000).

Stubbs, Kenneth Ray. *Erotic Passions: A Guide to Orgasmic Massage, Sensual Bathing, Oral Pleasuring.* (Tarcher, 2000).

Yeshe, Lama. *Introduction to Tantra: The Transformation of Desire.* (Wisdom Publications, 2001).

Videos

Ancient Secrets of Sexual Ecstasy—this video serves as a comprehensive guide to Tao and Tantric sexual techniques, including full-body orgasms and ejaculation control. It features leading Tantric experts and authors. Available at *www.sourcetantra.com.*

Best of Tantra DVD Set—this three-video set has lots of great information, and is priced at a discount over buying the items separately. Available at *www.sourcetantra.com*.

The Better Sex Guide to the Kama Sutra—another Sinclair Institute production, this video runs fifty minutes long and includes a bonus CD of sensual music. Real couples demonstrate positions from the Kama Sutra. Available at *www.amazon.com*.

Goddess Worship Video—this erotic video involves goddess worship and G-spot massage. Available at *www.GoddessTemple.com*.

Loving Sex: Ultimate Sensual Massage—this DVD offers very romantic and lush settings, and extremely sensual and erotic demonstrations. Available on *www.amazon.com*.

Sensual Couples Massage: Pleasure Your Woman and *Sensual Couples Massage: Pleasure Your Man*—these DVDs (sold separately) are each more than an hour long and demonstrate specific massage techniques designed to spice up your relationship. Available at *www.amazon.com*.

The Sensual Massage Kit: Massage for Men and Women—This two-video set tells (and shows) couples everything they need to know in order to treat their partner to the ultimate sensual massage. Available on *www.amazon.com*.

Tantra Massage for Lovers—this DVD set, which includes almost three hours of footage, features real-life couples demonstrating the art of sensual massage. Available at *www.amazon.com* and *www.ecstaticliving.com*.

The Tantric Guide to Better Sex—produced by Sinclair Intimacy Institute (a leader in relationship-oriented videos for adults), this DVD features sixty minutes of lovemaking tips and techniques related to prolonging orgasm, massage, and creating a romantic atmosphere, demonstrated by couples. Available at *www.amazon.com*.

Tantric Secrets of Sacred Sex—a classic Tantra film recently re-released on DVD. It features seventy-four minutes of Tantric techniques demonstrated by six real-life couples. Available on *www.tantra.com*.

Music

Language of Love: Music for the Kama Sutra, by Craig Pruess—relaxing music you can enjoy whether you are in the bedroom or not. This CD features many native Indian instruments and beautiful vocalizations. Available at *www.amazon.com*.

Lover's Lounge—featuring hypnotic melodies and pulsating beats from a variety of artists, this CD contains sixty minutes of sensual sounds that serve as a wonderful soundtrack to a sensual encounter. Available at *www.tantra.com*.

Tantra, by Anugama—this CD features music designed for meditation and introspection. Anugama's other selections include music for healing and exotic dance. Available at *www.amazon.com*.

Tantric Heart: Music for Lovers, by Shastro—this CD features forty-six minutes of sensual and soothing music, perfect for setting a romantic mood. Available at *www.tantra.com*.

Workshops

Bliss Tantra

✆Phone: (650) 323-4227

✐*www.blisstantra.com*

Courses (held in California) are taught by True Fellows, a certified massage therapist, hypnotherapist, and intuitive healer. She is also available to teach workshops at your location nationwide. Specific topics include sexual healing, intimate communication techniques, sacred sex, and full-body orgasms.

Cheryl Lazarus

✆Phone: (646) 584-9492

E-mail: *possibilitiescl@aol.com*

✐*www.spiritualpossibilities.com*

Cheryl Lazarus is a Tantra instructor and spiritual counselor who hosts full-day workshops and evening seminars for couples, where she teaches you how to create new pathways for sacred loving. Workshops are mainly held in the New York City area, but phone sessions are also available.

Four Freedoms Sacred Relationship

✆Phone: (800) 684-5308

E-mail: *4freedoms@tantraloving.com*

✐*www.tantra-sex.com*

This site, operated by Al Link and Pala Copeland, offers many opportunities to attend Tantra events, including an introductory weekend for couples new to Tantric techniques.

Institute for Ecstatic Living

✆Phone: (707) 987-3456

E-mail: *info@ecstaticliving.com*

✐*www.ecstaticliving.com*

This site offers Tantric workshops and vacations, including a Goddess Weekend just for women, and events specifically for singles. Teachers include Steve and Lokita Carter and Margot Anand.

Intimacy Retreats

✆Phone: (941) 349-6804

✐*www.intimacyretreats.com*

Workshop vacations for couples. Rekindle the passion in your relationship in a sexy, romantic setting. Workshops led by Richard and Diana Daffner, creators of Tantra Tai Chi and Lessons in Intimacy.

Lucy Becker Workshops

✆Phone: (416) 489-0557

E-mail: *lucy@tantraworkshops.com*

✐*www.tantraworkshops.com*

Lucy Becker is director of the Tantra Center of Toronto. She presents workshops designed to provide instruction in sexual skills and techniques ranging from beginner to advanced. Specific course topics include enhancing orgasm experiences, increasing the erotic energy in your relationship, and harnessing the power of an energy orgasm.

Sacred Loving

✆Phone: (800) 688-1715

E-mail: *niyaso@maui.net*

✐*www.SacredLoving.net*

Niyaso Carter, a native of India, has been guiding, teaching, and counseling individuals in the area of sacred sexuality for almost twenty years. She is the co-creator of the bestselling educational video *The Secrets of Sacred Sex*. She leads Tantric workshops and seminars, along with women-only retreats in Hawaii.

Tantra at Tahoe

✍ *www.tantraattahoe.com*

Private Tantra workshops featuring six-hour sessions of Tantra instruction, personalized to meet your individual needs and goals.

Tantra for Women

✆ Phone: (707) 824-1118

✍ *www.tantraforwomen.com*

Tantric workshops and events, most of which are for women only, held in California.

TantraQuest

✆ Phone: (808) 345-0570

✍ *www.tantraquest.com*

Tantra workshops and retreats (based in Hawaii; also hosts events in Canada and other locations).

International Workshops

Australia

The Australian School of Tantra

E-mail: *info@australianschooloftantra.com.au*

✍ *http://australianschooloftantra.com.au*

Australian service offering workshops (including women-only events), home courses, and private sessions.

Czech Republic

International Tantric Courses in Prague

E-mail: *institut@tantra.cz*

✍ *www.tantra.cz/tantricworkshops*

Presented by Tantra Institute CZ, workshops held in Czech with simultaneous translations in English.

England

Butterfly Workshops

E-mail: *info@butterflyworkshops.com*

✍ *www.butterflyworkshops.com*

Workshops help monthly in the London area.

Index

The EVERYTHING Series!

BUSINESS & PERSONAL FINANCE

Everything® Accounting Book
Everything® Budgeting Book
Everything® Business Planning Book
Everything® Coaching and Mentoring Book
Everything® Fundraising Book
Everything® Get Out of Debt Book
Everything® Grant Writing Book
Everything® Guide to Personal Finance for Single Mothers
Everything® Home-Based Business Book, 2nd Ed.
Everything® Homebuying Book, 2nd Ed.
Everything® Homeselling Book, 2nd Ed.
Everything® Improve Your Credit Book
Everything® Investing Book, 2nd Ed.
Everything® Landlording Book
Everything® Leadership Book
Everything® Managing People Book, 2nd Ed.
Everything® Negotiating Book
Everything® Online Auctions Book
Everything® Online Business Book
Everything® Personal Finance Book
Everything® Personal Finance in Your 20s and 30s Book
Everything® Project Management Book
Everything® Real Estate Investing Book
Everything® Retirement Planning Book
Everything® Robert's Rules Book, $7.95
Everything® Selling Book
Everything® Start Your Own Business Book, 2nd Ed.
Everything® Wills & Estate Planning Book

COOKING

Everything® Barbecue Cookbook
Everything® Bartender's Book, $9.95
Everything® Cheese Book
Everything® Chinese Cookbook
Everything® Classic Recipes Book
Everything® Cocktail Parties and Drinks Book
Everything® College Cookbook
Everything® Cooking for Baby and Toddler Book
Everything® Cooking for Two Cookbook
Everything® Diabetes Cookbook
Everything® Easy Gourmet Cookbook
Everything® Fondue Cookbook
Everything® Fondue Party Book
Everything® Gluten-Free Cookbook
Everything® Glycemic Index Cookbook
Everything® Grilling Cookbook

Everything® Healthy Meals in Minutes Cookbook
Everything® Holiday Cookbook
Everything® Indian Cookbook
Everything® Italian Cookbook
Everything® Low-Carb Cookbook
Everything® Low-Fat High-Flavor Cookbook
Everything® Low-Salt Cookbook
Everything® Meals for a Month Cookbook
Everything® Mediterranean Cookbook
Everything® Mexican Cookbook
Everything® No Trans Fat Cookbook
Everything® One-Pot Cookbook
Everything® Pizza Cookbook
Everything® Quick and Easy 30-Minute, 5-Ingredient Cookbook
Everything® Quick Meals Cookbook
Everything® Slow Cooker Cookbook
Everything® Slow Cooking for a Crowd Cookbook
Everything® Soup Cookbook
Everything® Stir-Fry Cookbook
Everything® Tex-Mex Cookbook
Everything® Thai Cookbook
Everything® Vegetarian Cookbook
Everything® Wild Game Cookbook
Everything® Wine Book, 2nd Ed.

GAMES

Everything® 15-Minute Sudoku Book, $9.95
Everything® 30-Minute Sudoku Book, $9.95
Everything® Blackjack Strategy Book
Everything® Brain Strain Book, $9.95
Everything® Bridge Book
Everything® Card Games Book
Everything® Card Tricks Book, $9.95
Everything® Casino Gambling Book, 2nd Ed.
Everything® Chess Basics Book
Everything® Craps Strategy Book
Everything® Crossword and Puzzle Book
Everything® Crossword Challenge Book
Everything® Crosswords for the Beach Book, $9.95
Everything® Cryptograms Book, $9.95
Everything® Easy Crosswords Book
Everything® Easy Kakuro Book, $9.95
Everything® Easy Large Print Crosswords Book
Everything® Games Book, 2nd Ed.
Everything® Giant Sudoku Book, $9.95
Everything® Kakuro Challenge Book, $9.95
Everything® Large-Print Crossword Challenge Book

Everything® Large-Print Crosswords Book
Everything® Lateral Thinking Puzzles Book, $9.95
Everything® Mazes Book
Everything® Movie Crosswords Book, $9.95
Everything® Online Poker Book, $12.95
Everything® Pencil Puzzles Book, $9.95
Everything® Poker Strategy Book
Everything® Pool & Billiards Book
Everything® Sports Crosswords Book, $9.95
Everything® Test Your IQ Book, $9.95
Everything® Texas Hold 'Em Book, $9.95
Everything® Travel Crosswords Book, $9.95
Everything® Word Games Challenge Book
Everything® Word Scramble Book
Everything® Word Search Book

HEALTH

Everything® Alzheimer's Book
Everything® Diabetes Book
Everything® Health Guide to Adult Bipolar Disorder
Everything® Health Guide to Controlling Anxiety
Everything® Health Guide to Fibromyalgia
Everything® Health Guide to Postpartum Care
Everything® Health Guide to Thyroid Disease
Everything® Hypnosis Book
Everything® Low Cholesterol Book
Everything® Massage Book
Everything® Menopause Book
Everything® Nutrition Book
Everything® Reflexology Book
Everything® Stress Management Book

HISTORY

Everything® American Government Book
Everything® American History Book, 2nd Ed.
Everything® Civil War Book
Everything® Freemasons Book
Everything® Irish History & Heritage Book
Everything® Middle East Book

HOBBIES

Everything® Candlemaking Book
Everything® Cartooning Book
Everything® Coin Collecting Book
Everything® Drawing Book
Everything® Family Tree Book, 2nd Ed.
Everything® Knitting Book
Everything® Knots Book
Everything® Photography Book

Everything® Quilting Book
Everything® Scrapbooking Book
Everything® Sewing Book
Everything® Soapmaking Book, 2nd Ed.
Everything® Woodworking Book

HOME IMPROVEMENT

Everything® Feng Shui Book
Everything® Feng Shui Decluttering Book, $9.95
Everything® Fix-It Book
Everything® Home Decorating Book
Everything® Home Storage Solutions Book
Everything® Homebuilding Book
Everything® Organize Your Home Book

KIDS' BOOKS

All titles are $7.95

Everything® Kids' Animal Puzzle & Activity Book
Everything® Kids' Baseball Book, 4th Ed.
Everything® Kids' Bible Trivia Book
Everything® Kids' Bugs Book
Everything® Kids' Cars and Trucks Puzzle
& Activity Book
Everything® Kids' Christmas Puzzle
& Activity Book
Everything® Kids' Cookbook
Everything® Kids' Crazy Puzzles Book
Everything® Kids' Dinosaurs Book
Everything® Kids' First Spanish Puzzle and
Activity Book
Everything® Kids' Gross Cookbook
Everything® Kids' Gross Hidden Pictures Book
Everything® Kids' Gross Jokes Book
Everything® Kids' Gross Mazes Book
Everything® Kids' Gross Puzzle and
Activity Book
Everything® Kids' Halloween Puzzle
& Activity Book
Everything® Kids' Hidden Pictures Book
Everything® Kids' Horses Book
Everything® Kids' Joke Book
Everything® Kids' Knock Knock Book
Everything® Kids' Learning Spanish Book
Everything® Kids' Math Puzzles Book
Everything® Kids' Mazes Book
Everything® Kids' Money Book
Everything® Kids' Nature Book
Everything® Kids' Pirates Puzzle and Activity Book
Everything® Kids' Presidents Book
Everything® Kids' Princess Puzzle and Activity Book
Everything® Kids' Puzzle Book
Everything® Kids' Riddles & Brain Teasers Book
Everything® Kids' Science Experiments Book
Everything® Kids' Sharks Book
Everything® Kids' Soccer Book
Everything® Kids' States Book
Everything® Kids' Travel Activity Book

KIDS' STORY BOOKS

Everything® Fairy Tales Book

LANGUAGE

Everything® Conversational Japanese Book with
CD, $19.95
Everything® French Grammar Book
Everything® French Phrase Book, $9.95
Everything® French Verb Book, $9.95
Everything® German Practice Book with CD,
$19.95
Everything® Inglés Book
**Everything® Intermediate Spanish Book with
CD, $19.95**
**Everything® Learning Brazilian Portuguese
Book with CD, $19.95**
Everything® Learning French Book
Everything® Learning German Book
Everything® Learning Italian Book
Everything® Learning Latin Book
**Everything® Learning Spanish Book with
CD, 2nd Edition, $19.95**
Everything® Russian Practice Book with CD, $19.95
Everything® Sign Language Book
Everything® Spanish Grammar Book
Everything® Spanish Phrase Book, $9.95
Everything® Spanish Practice Book
with CD, $19.95
Everything® Spanish Verb Book, $9.95
Everything® Speaking Mandarin Chinese Book
with CD, $19.95

MUSIC

Everything® Drums Book with CD, $19.95
**Everything® Guitar Book with CD, 2nd
Edition, $19.95**
Everything® Guitar Chords Book with CD, $19.95
Everything® Home Recording Book
Everything® Music Theory Book with CD, $19.95
Everything® Reading Music Book with CD, $19.95
Everything® Rock & Blues Guitar Book
with CD, $19.95
**Everything® Rock and Blues Piano Book
with CD, $19.95**
Everything® Songwriting Book

NEW AGE

Everything® Astrology Book, 2nd Ed.
Everything® Birthday Personology Book
Everything® Dreams Book, 2nd Ed.
Everything® Love Signs Book, $9.95
Everything® Numerology Book
Everything® Paganism Book
Everything® Palmistry Book
Everything® Psychic Book
Everything® Reiki Book

Everything® Sex Signs Book, $9.95
Everything® Tarot Book, 2nd Ed.
Everything® Toltec Wisdom Book
Everything® Wicca and Witchcraft Book

PARENTING

Everything® Baby Names Book, 2nd Ed.
Everything® Baby Shower Book
Everything® Baby's First Year Book
Everything® Birthing Book
Everything® Breastfeeding Book
Everything® Father-to-Be Book
Everything® Father's First Year Book
Everything® Get Ready for Baby Book
Everything® Get Your Baby to Sleep Book, $9.95
Everything® Getting Pregnant Book
Everything® Guide to Raising a One-Year-Old
Everything® Guide to Raising a Two-Year-Old
Everything® Homeschooling Book
Everything® Mother's First Year Book
**Everything® Parent's Guide to Childhood
Illnesses**
Everything® Parent's Guide to Children
and Divorce
Everything® Parent's Guide to Children
with ADD/ADHD
Everything® Parent's Guide to Children
with Asperger's Syndrome
Everything® Parent's Guide to Children
with Autism
Everything® Parent's Guide to Children with
Bipolar Disorder
**Everything® Parent's Guide to Children with
Depression**
Everything® Parent's Guide to Children
with Dyslexia
**Everything® Parent's Guide to Children with
Juvenile Diabetes**
Everything® Parent's Guide to Positive Discipline
Everything® Parent's Guide to Raising a
Successful Child
Everything® Parent's Guide to Raising Boys
Everything® Parent's Guide to Raising Girls
Everything® Parent's Guide to Raising Siblings
Everything® Parent's Guide to Sensory
Integration Disorder
Everything® Parent's Guide to Tantrums
Everything® Parent's Guide to the Strong-Willed
Child
Everything® Parenting a Teenager Book
Everything® Potty Training Book, $9.95
Everything® Pregnancy Book, 3rd Ed.
Everything® Pregnancy Fitness Book
Everything® Pregnancy Nutrition Book
Everything® Pregnancy Organizer, 2nd Ed., $16.95
Everything® Toddler Activities Book
Everything® Toddler Book

Everything® Tween Book
Everything® Twins, Triplets, and More Book

PETS

Everything® Aquarium Book
Everything® Boxer Book
Everything® Cat Book, 2nd Ed.
Everything® Chihuahua Book
Everything® Dachshund Book
Everything® Dog Book
Everything® Dog Health Book
Everything® Dog Obedience Book
Everything® Dog Owner's Organizer, $16.95
Everything® Dog Training and Tricks Book
Everything® German Shepherd Book
Everything® Golden Retriever Book
Everything® Horse Book
Everything® Horse Care Book
Everything® Horseback Riding Book
Everything® Labrador Retriever Book
Everything® Poodle Book
Everything® Pug Book
Everything® Puppy Book
Everything® Rottweiler Book
Everything® Small Dogs Book
Everything® Tropical Fish Book
Everything® Yorkshire Terrier Book

REFERENCE

Everything® American Presidents Book
Everything® Blogging Book
Everything® Build Your Vocabulary Book
Everything® Car Care Book
Everything® Classical Mythology Book
Everything® Da Vinci Book
Everything® Divorce Book
Everything® Einstein Book
Everything® Enneagram Book
Everything® Etiquette Book, 2nd Ed.
Everything® Inventions and Patents Book
Everything® Mafia Book
Everything® Philosophy Book
Everything® Pirates Book
Everything® Psychology Book

RELIGION

Everything® Angels Book
Everything® Bible Book
Everything® Buddhism Book
Everything® Catholicism Book
Everything® Christianity Book
Everything® Gnostic Gospels Book
Everything® History of the Bible Book
Everything® Jesus Book

Everything® Jewish History & Heritage Book
Everything® Judaism Book
Everything® Kabbalah Book
Everything® Koran Book
Everything® Mary Book
Everything® Mary Magdalene Book
Everything® Prayer Book
Everything® Saints Book, 2nd Ed.
Everything® Torah Book
Everything® Understanding Islam Book
Everything® World's Religions Book
Everything® Zen Book

SCHOOL & CAREERS

Everything® Alternative Careers Book
Everything® Career Tests Book
Everything® College Major Test Book
Everything® College Survival Book, 2nd Ed.
Everything® Cover Letter Book, 2nd Ed.
Everything® Filmmaking Book
Everything® Get-a-Job Book, 2nd Ed.
Everything® Guide to Being a Paralegal
Everything® Guide to Being a Personal Trainer
Everything® Guide to Being a Real Estate Agent
Everything® Guide to Being a Sales Rep
Everything® Guide to Careers in Health Care
Everything® Guide to Careers in Law Enforcement
Everything® Guide to Government Jobs
Everything® Guide to Starting and Running a Restaurant
Everything® Job Interview Book
Everything® New Nurse Book
Everything® New Teacher Book
Everything® Paying for College Book
Everything® Practice Interview Book
Everything® Resume Book, 2nd Ed.
Everything® Study Book

SELF-HELP

Everything® Dating Book, 2nd Ed.
Everything® Great Sex Book
Everything® Self-Esteem Book
Everything® Tantric Sex Book

SPORTS & FITNESS

Everything® Easy Fitness Book
Everything® Running Book
Everything® Weight Training Book

TRAVEL

Everything® Family Guide to Cruise Vacations
Everything® Family Guide to Hawaii
Everything® Family Guide to Las Vegas, 2nd Ed.
Everything® Family Guide to Mexico
Everything® Family Guide to New York City, 2nd Ed.
Everything® Family Guide to RV Travel & Campgrounds
Everything® Family Guide to the Caribbean
Everything® Family Guide to the Walt Disney World Resort®, Universal Studios®, and Greater Orlando, 4th Ed.
Everything® Family Guide to Timeshares
Everything® Family Guide to Washington D.C., 2nd Ed.

WEDDINGS

Everything® Bachelorette Party Book, $9.95
Everything® Bridesmaid Book, $9.95
Everything® Destination Wedding Book
Everything® Elopement Book, $9.95
Everything® Father of the Bride Book, $9.95
Everything® Groom Book, $9.95
Everything® Mother of the Bride Book, $9.95
Everything® Outdoor Wedding Book
Everything® Wedding Book, 3rd Ed.
Everything® Wedding Checklist, $9.95
Everything® Wedding Etiquette Book, $9.95
Everything® Wedding Organizer, 2nd Ed., $16.95
Everything® Wedding Shower Book, $9.95
Everything® Wedding Vows Book, $9.95
Everything® Wedding Workout Book
Everything® Weddings on a Budget Book, $9.95

WRITING

Everything® Creative Writing Book
Everything® Get Published Book, 2nd Ed.
Everything® Grammar and Style Book
Everything® Guide to Magazine Writing
Everything® Guide to Writing a Book Proposal
Everything® Guide to Writing a Novel
Everything® Guide to Writing Children's Books
Everything® Guide to Writing Copy
Everything® Guide to Writing Research Papers
Everything® Screenwriting Book
Everything® Writing Poetry Book
Everything® Writing Well Book